Redirecting Alzheimer Strategy - Tracing Memory Loss to Self Pathology

Edited by Denis Larrivee

Published in London, United Kingdom

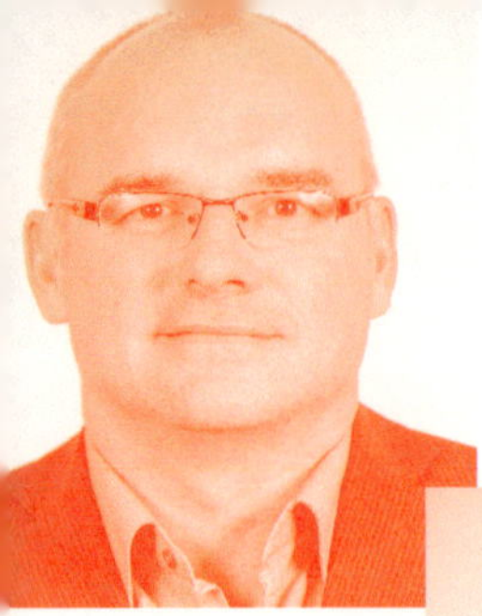
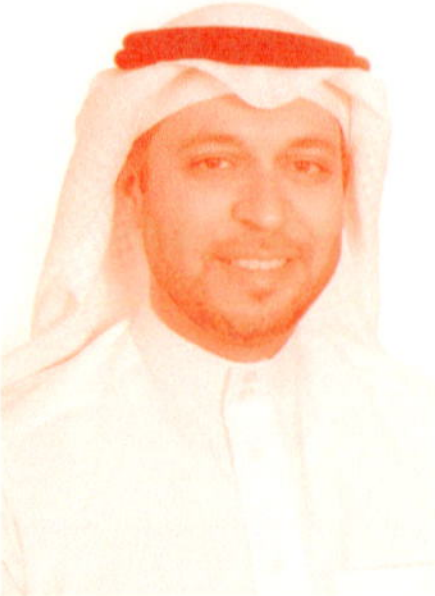
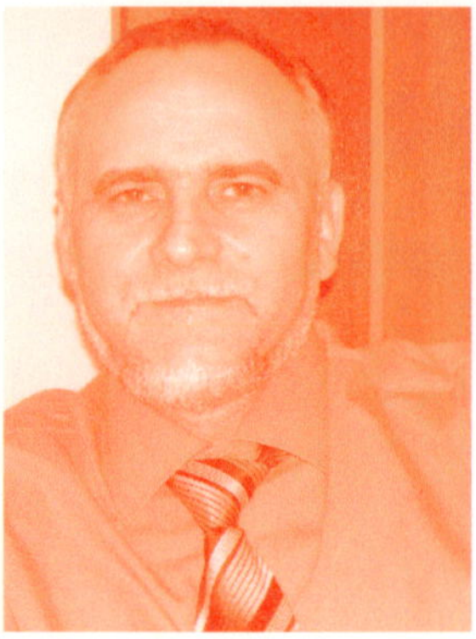
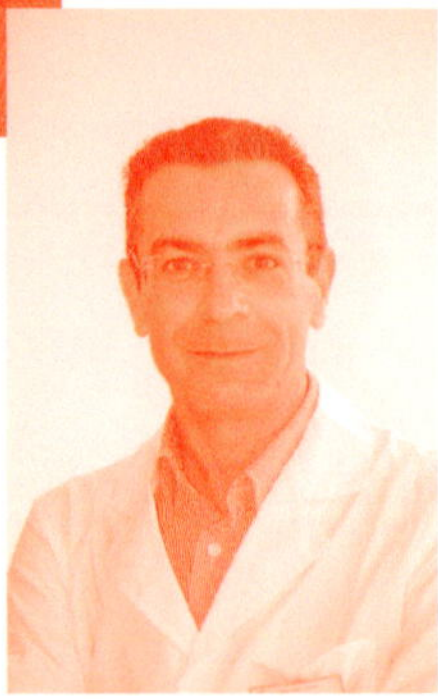
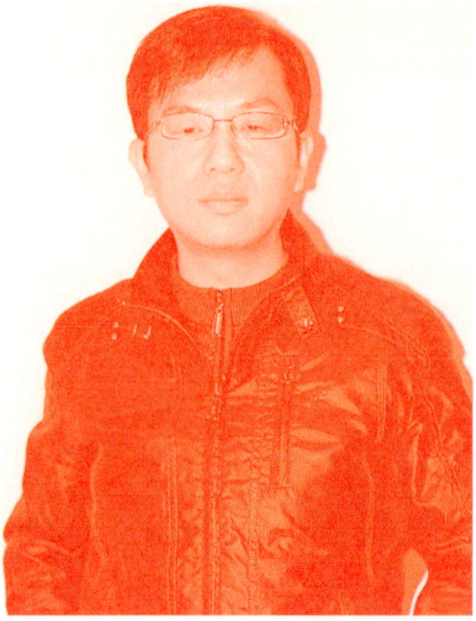
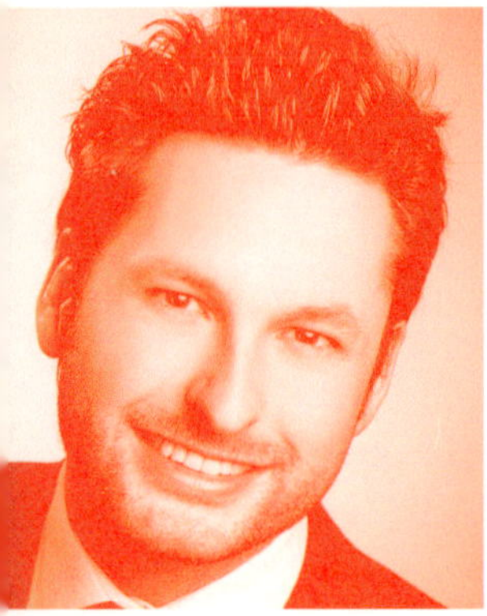
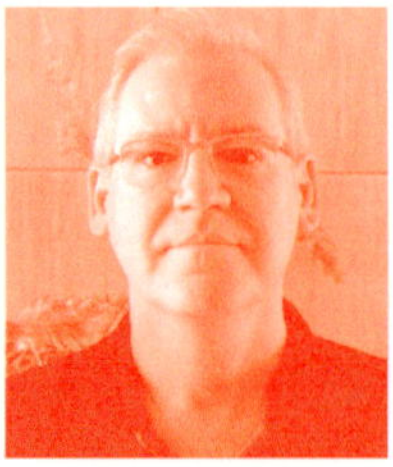

IntechOpen

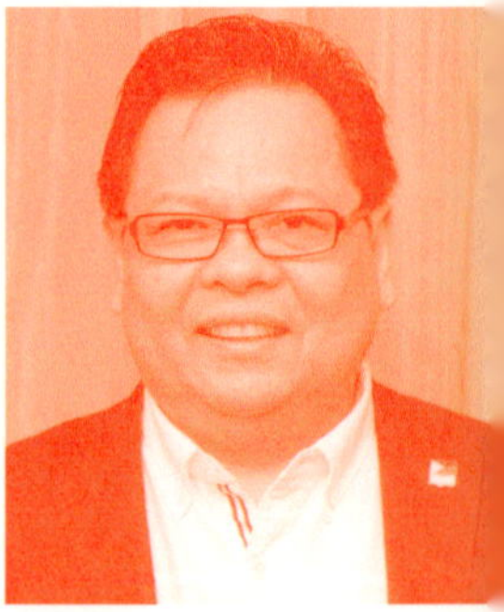
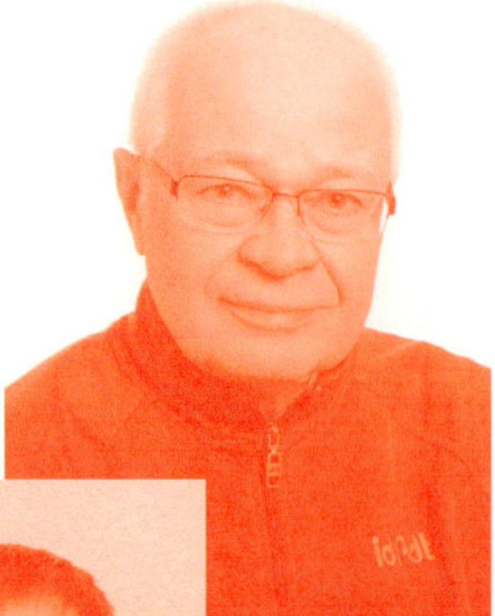
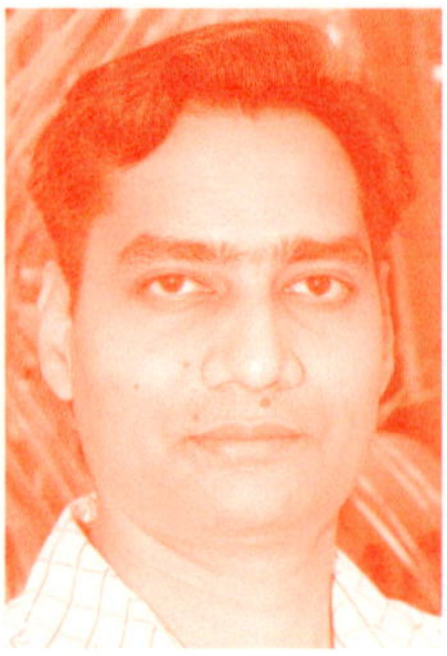
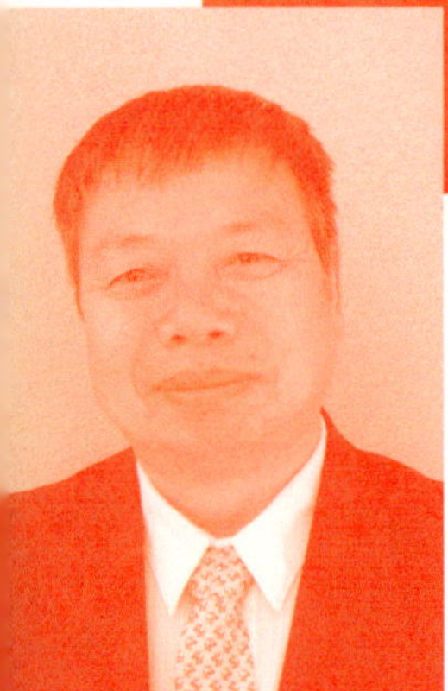
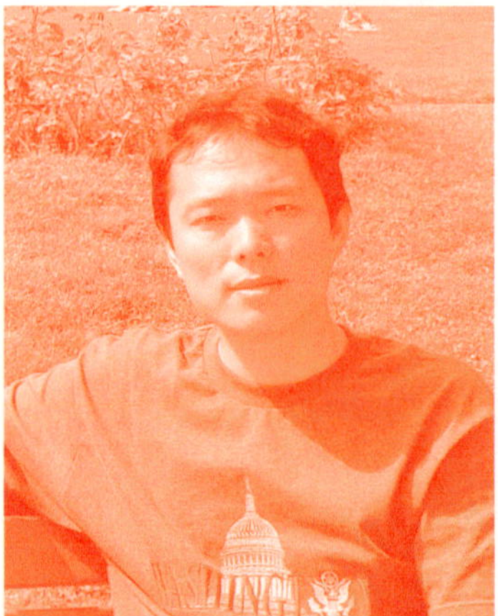
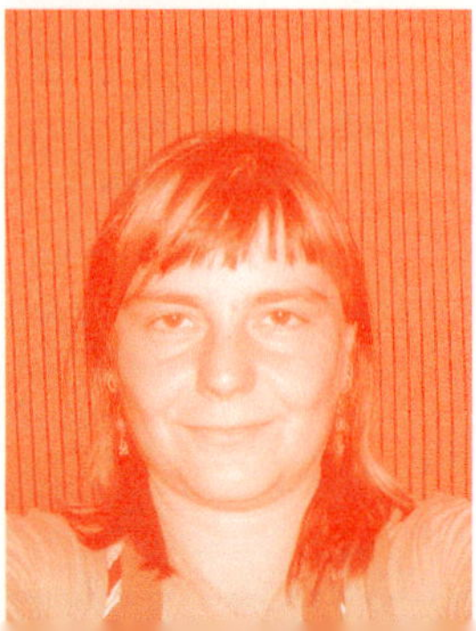

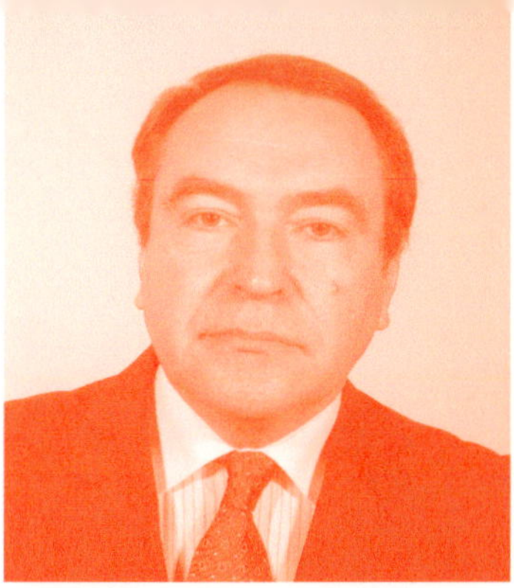
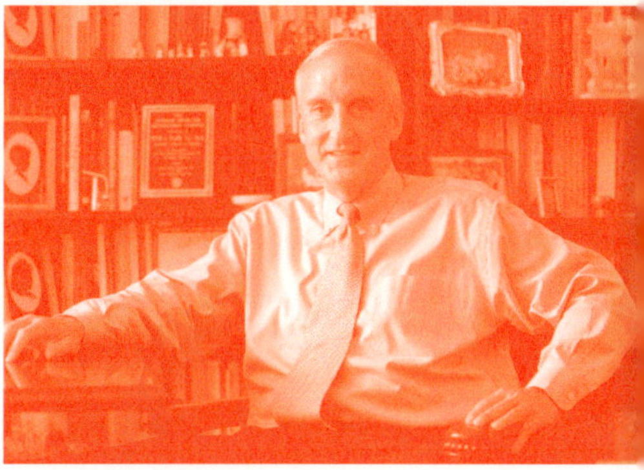
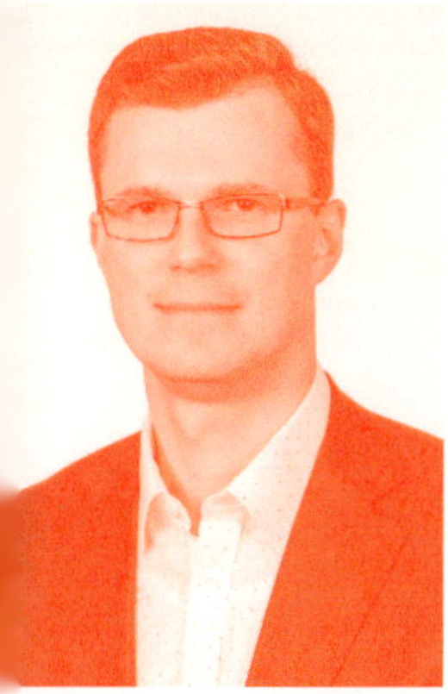
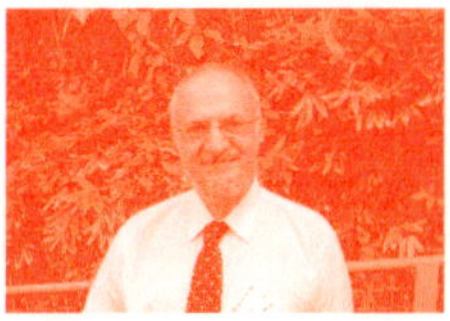
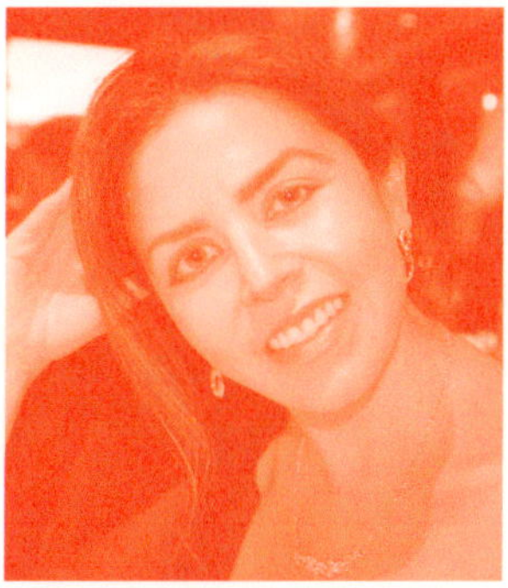

Supporting open minds since 2005

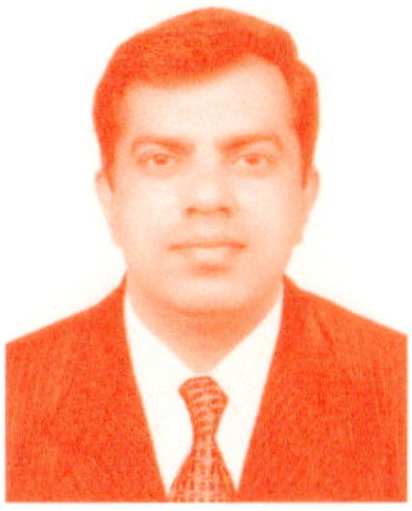
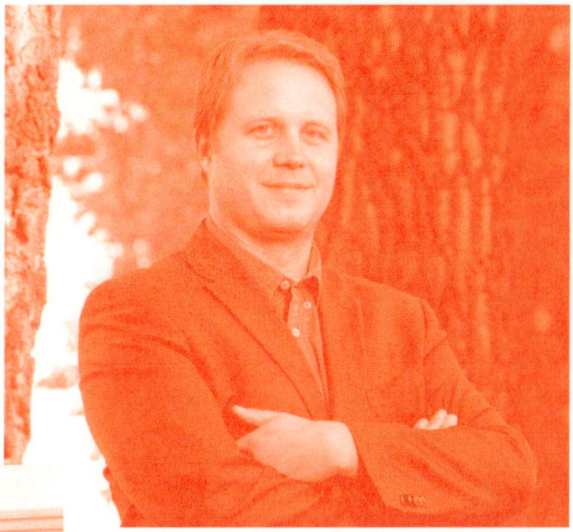
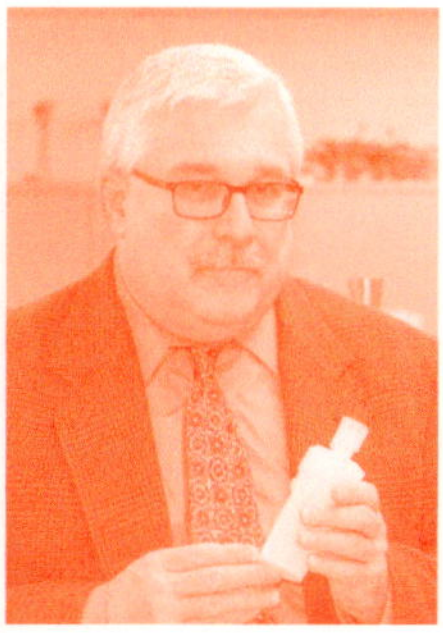
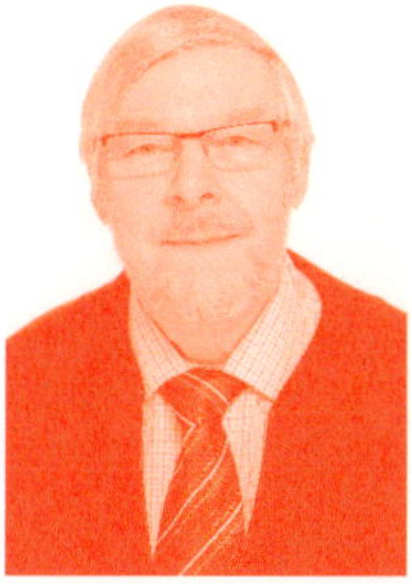
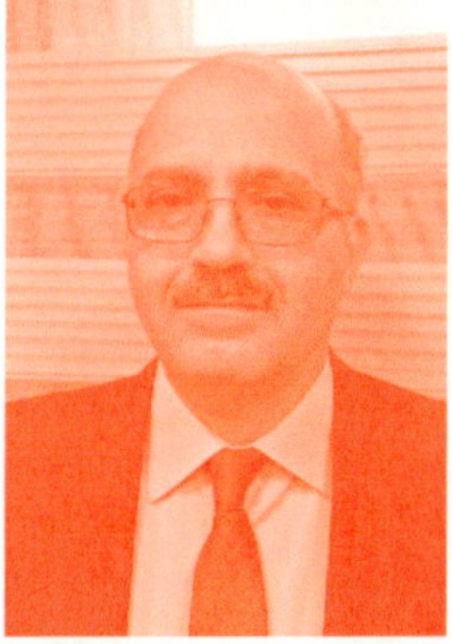
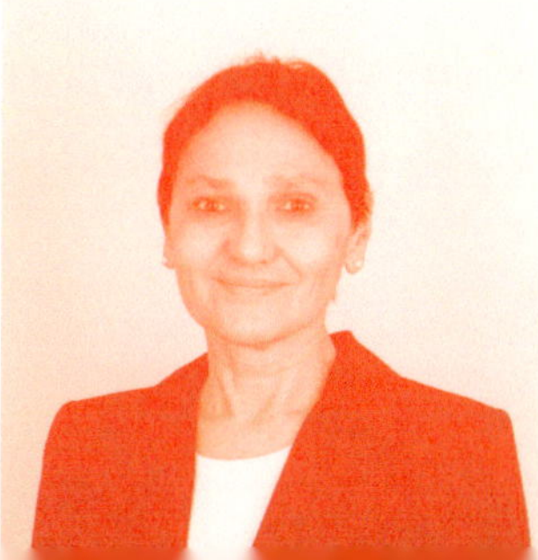
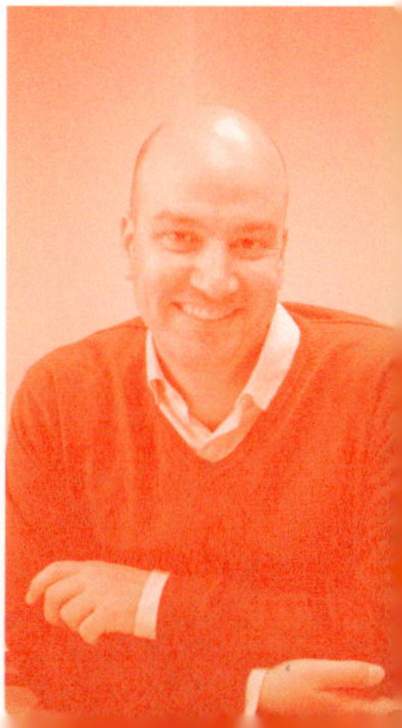

Redirecting Alzheimer Strategy - Tracing Memory Loss to Self Pathology
http://dx.doi.org/10.5772/intechopen.77687
Edited by Denis Larrivee

Contributors
Winnie Sun, Srija Biswas, Ping Zou, Michelle Dacanay, José V. Pardo, Bilqees Bano, Fakhra Amin, Terezia Fertalova, Iveta Ondriova, Francisco Javier Garzón-Maldonado, María Dolores Martinez-Valle Torres, Stavros J. Baloyannis, Denis Larrivee

First published in London, United Kingdom, 2019 by IntechOpen
IntechOpen is the global imprint of INTECHOPEN LIMITED, registered in England and Wales, registration number: 11086078, The Shard, 25th floor, 32 London Bridge Street
London, SE19SG – United Kingdom
Printed in Croatia

British Library Cataloguing-in-Publication Data
A catalogue record for this book is available from the British Library

Additional hard and PDF copies can be obtained from orders@intechopen.com

Redirecting Alzheimer Strategy - Tracing Memory Loss to Self Pathology
Edited by Denis Larrivee
p. cm.
Print ISBN 978-1-78984-009-4
Online ISBN 978-1-78984-010-0
eBook (PDF) ISBN 978-1-83962-210-6

For EU product safety concerns:
IN TECH d.o.o., Prolaz Marije Krucifikse Kozulić 3, 51000 Rijeka, Croatia, info@intechopen.com or visit our website at intechopen.com.

Meet the editor

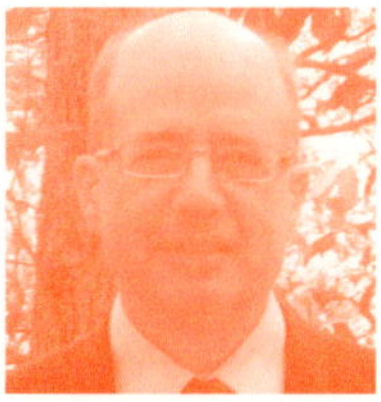

Dr. Denis Larrivee is a visiting scholar at the Mind and Brain Institute, University of Navarra Medical School and Loyola University, Chicago, and has held professorships at Weill Cornell University Medical College, NYC, and Purdue University, Indiana. A former fellow at Yale University's Medical School he received the Association for Research in Vision and Ophthalmology's first place award for studies on photoreceptor degenerative and developmental mechanisms. He is the editor of a recently released text on brain computer interfacing with IntechOpen Publishing and an editorial board member of the journals *Annals of Neurology and Neurological Sciences* (USA) and *EC Neurology* (UK). An International Neuroethics Society expert he is the author of more than 75 papers and book chapters on such varied journals/venues as *Neurology and Neurological Sciences* (USA), *Journal of Neuroscience*, *Journal of Religion and Mental Health*, and *IEEE Explore*. In 2018 he was a finalist in the international Joseph Ratzinger Expanded Reason award.

Contents

Preface

It is fair to say that no brain disease occupies more research study today than Alzheimer's disease (AD). Among the many excellent reasons for this circumstance are the bleak prognosis and relentless progression; large cohorts of baby boomers entering an age of greatly increased cognitive risk; spectacular advances in medical care that have prolonged lifespan; and ever-mounting risk with age. Moreover, there is perhaps no dearer feature than self-awareness and the memory of self across time, all of which are taken as the disease marks its course.

Often unattributed in propelling interest in AD is the success of the research enterprise that has advanced the understanding of the brain. From Hodgkin and Huxley's characterization of the action potential less than 70 years ago, neuroscience has identified nearly all brain neurotransmitters, resolved the structure of the major ion channels, and stands poised to decipher the operations of hundreds of thousands of neurons in joint activity. The product of the scientific method of these successes have instilled a confidence that disease causes will ultimately succumb to the persistence of research, and that the accumulation of data from appropriately designed experiments will blossom into therapies that will arrest and perhaps even reverse AD. Such confidence is being tested, however, and may be prolonged by the very strategies that repeat the premises of the past research methods that have so successfully propelled other aspects of neuroscientific research.

Despite the decades of intense research and a rising wave of elderly people, AD remains poorly understood, an enigma amid a tide of neuroscientific advance. Identified more than a century ago, AD is characterized by a constellation of cognitive dysfunctions, the earliest and most prominent being that of impaired recollection. In its many decades of investigation, numerous theories have sought to unify AD's disparate symptoms within a common causal frame. Current readings list some 13 influential hypotheses, the most widely invoked involving the biomarkers, β-amyloid plaques, and neurofibrillary tangles, identified by Alois Alzheimer more than 100 years ago. Other frequently cited causes include dysfunctional energy resourcing, with evidence pointing toward either glycolytic or electron transport stages.

The mystery of AD's origin is compounded by the genetic observations intended to provide improved predictive diagnosis for a swelling demographic sector. Its set of risk alleles is large by non-cognitive disease standards, and new alleles are regularly being added. The current membership is highly diverse, with some alleles affecting the early onset phase, such as the presenilin genes, the late-phase β-amyloid protein, lipidogenesis genes, and even cytoskeletal and immune genes, among a growing set. Most alleles display small phenotypic effects that are non-Mendelian with low penetrance and that are of a quantitative rather than a qualitative nature. Overall, the relatively small effects of individual alleles and the large field of membership obscure rather than enlighten, offering meager insight into the causal factors inducing AD's relentless progression. Indeed, genetic observations suggest that affected gene products are neither individually crucial nor functionally irreplaceable components of cognitive processes. They suggest instead that while exerting a limited influence on individual constituents, AD's chief effects may instead target systemic and even global events, where cognition is the product of more flexible physical associations, and where the dysfunction of individual components does little to diminish functional adequacy.

> *What the inconclusive results thus appear to do is call into question an understanding of cognition that views it from the bottom up—the study of which is eminently suited by the scientific method—and that dispenses with a philosophy of biology concerned with how organismal properties operate, for which cognition is the medium.*

Accordingly, the chapters of this text intend to give evidence that "bottom-up" approaches—nearly exclusively pursued in AD research—yield limited insight into causal etiology and so implicate the need to undertake fundamentally different strategic avenues. Chapter 2, for example, is illustrative for showing how singular theories like that of impaired glycolysis face numerous findings that conflict with outcomes predicted by theory, as does Chapter 3 on mitochondrial dysfunction. Chapter 4 proposes, in consequence, that protective measures against cellular lysis may offer a general though non-specific way forward to arresting degeneration. The question of whether the findings obtained from these studies are etiological, or merely epiphenomenal, accordingly remain unaddressed. Indeed, a number of studies point to impairments of global phenomena, like the self-construct, in AD. Recent findings, for example, have demonstrated that functional connectivities between key nuclei within the default mode network, a domain linked to self-recognition, are weakened. Relating these specific global effects to the sort of generalized disarray that is seen at lower levels of function suggests that old strategies used for exploring the disease would be better directed in new strategical ventures concerned with global cognition, a point emphasized in the first chapter for looking beyond reductive approaches alone.

A significant issue also raised by the present lack of insight into etiology is that of determining patient therapy for what is manifestly a debilitating and personally tragic circumstance. Extant findings from a large body of research suggest that treatment options relying on the correction of single molecular entities are likely to offer little that will be therapeutically advantageous or substantially mitigate the advance of the disease. In the absence of such singular pharmacological options, they suggest that therapies ordered to global aspects of cognition are likely to be more fruitful in slowing symptomatic progression. In this vein, widely adopted healthcare management models, discussed in Chapters 5 and 6 that emphasize the person as a whole, are more likely to improve global self-representation through cognitive integration. As pointed out in Chapter 7 on the current level of cultural diversity within immigrant populations, these efforts will need to be expanded to enable the access of these groups to such care, particularly in cases where cultural constraints impede involvement.

It is hoped that this text will inspire debate on new “top-down” strategical alternatives to the current preeminent “bottom-up” models and underscore the humanitarian issue that is at the heart of care for the AD patient.

Denis Larrivee
Visiting Scholar,
Loyola University Chicago,
USA

Mind and Brain Group
University of Navarra Medical School,
Pamplona, Spain

Section 1

Thematic Issues in Modern Alzheimer Research

Chapter 1

Introductory Chapter: Beyond Risk Alleles - Invoking Cognitive Lesions in Top-Down Strategic Analysis

Denis Larrivee

1. Introduction

Improvements in medical care have significantly extended life expectancies, upwardly shifting demographic indicators of the elderly worldwide. Coupled with falling birth rates, however, the number of patients suffering cognitive deficits has also increased. World Health Organization projections, for example, indicate that by 2050, more than 20% will fall in this sector, with considerably higher percentages in developed nations, placing large numbers of individuals at risk [1]. Among the elderly the most prevalent neurodegenerative disease is Alzheimer's disease (AD) with a lifetime risk above 60 of 33% for males and 45% for females. Its growth rate is anticipated to exceed nearly 100% that of current levels in developed nations and more than 300% in Southeast Asian countries [2]. These increases in age-related diseases, moreover, add to an already significant burden from such prevalent mental health diseases as schizophrenia and bipolar disorder.

Symptomatically, prevalent diseases like AD and Korsakoff's syndrome, exhibit profound memory losses. In AD a broad consensus posits that its early symptoms include memory lapses that involve episodic memory, semantic recall, and visual orienting [3]. Among its earliest is an impaired sense of smell, a feature that may relate to evolutionary survival value. With the progression of AD, recent memories fade, and there is a proportionately greater retention of older ones, a characteristic observation termed Ribot's law.

Defined as a process of encoding, storing, and retrieving sensorial or mental information, memory dysfunctions induced by AD may be functionally interpreted as to the manner by which one or more of these phases are affected. Accordingly, the loss of formed memories, or retrograde amnesia, observed in AD patients, can be explained either by a loss of stored memories or an inability to retrieve them. In fact, existing evidence suggests that both phases are affected. Anatomical studies, for example, show a deterioration of thinly myelinated regions like the hippocampus relatively early in the disease progression compared to other regions [4]. Since the hippocampus is a critical center for recently formed memories, this evidence is consistent with loss of memories, particularly those that have formed first.

On the other hand, the disease is known to also specifically affect DMN operation [5], a domain thought to be critical to forming the self-construct. First identified by nuclear imaging studies that showed consistently higher levels of activity during passive task conditions, the DMN was hypothesized to monitor the external environment, body, and even emotions [6]. Task-related increases in activity in regional brain zones coincided with its decreased activity, indicating a reciprocal relation between the two zones related to the performance state of the

IntechOpen

task. Functional MRI shows that these relative activity levels are substantially and progressively altered by Alzheimer's disease [7]. For example, in AD patients the posterior cingulate and right inferior temporal cortical activities decline, whereas the activity of the bilateral inferior parietal cortex increases. Because the zones form central connectivity hubs within the DMN, the activity changes appear to reflect a weakening of causally influential relations among its principal nuclei. Metastability indices for AD patients, for example, are reduced in decoupled, desynchronized states, revealing that the disease progression significantly reduces the brain's ability to entrain regional dynamical activity [8].

Unlike AD, on the other hand, Korsakoff's syndrome manifests as a persistent memory impairment that associates chiefly with the acquisition of new information [9–12]. Accordingly, it has been frequently classified as a disease yielding an anterograde form of amnesia. Like AD, on the other hand, its influence is multipronged, with studies showing that it also affects memory retrieval. Moreover, other studies show a preponderance of perifunctional influences rather than direct influences on episodic and semantic memory per se. For example, context memory, which makes an important contribution to memory recollection, has been shown to be significantly impaired in Korsakoff's patient. In memory tests, additionally, differential impairments are seen between AD and Korsakoff's disease and also Huntingdon's disease. For example, KS and HD patients performed considerably better than AD patients in recall memory [13].

The complexity of the influences of the two diseases on memory, notwithstanding, the distinctions in their manifestation suggest that these could be exploited both to resolve the likely etiological differences between the two and also to gain insight into underlying processes of memory and its relation to the self-construct. Differences in phenotypic manifestation, notably, have motivated much research, on the presupposition that they reflect the presence of different processes contributing to a single, albeit complex, function. Moreover, differences in manifestation also have bearing on therapeutic interventions and managed patient care, illustrated in the chapters of this edited volume.

Research into diseases like hemophilia has traditionally sought to resolve underlying etiopathological features by exploring genetic and biochemical differences that traced their manifestations to single, albeit critical, constituents of biochemical mechanisms, like the coagulation defects of Factor VIII in hemophiliac patients [14]. Cognitive diseases, on the other hand, are likely to differ greatly from those with such 'metabolite-like features due to the nervous systems's global role in integrating organismal function. Thus numerous aspects affected by these diseases are likely to differ, including their manner of functioning, composition, and hierarchy [15, 16]. Hence, there is the question of whether traditional strategies based on reductive approaches that attempt to determine etiology from genetic or molecular origins are an adequate beginning for investigating normal or disease-affected cognition. Indeed, the present volume illustrates both the challenge and the enigmatic character of such diseases. Accordingly, it is the intention of this introductory chapter to consider the limitations to study emerging from the adoption of such reductive strategies and the prospects of exploiting "higher-order differences" of the sort seen in AD and Korsakoff's disease, to infer etiopathological origins.

2. Approaching etiology through risk alleles

Clinically, the identification of risk alleles has significantly benefitted medical diagnosis and therapy. For example, diagnosis of the risk allele for hemophilia A, Factor VIII has high predictive power of, for example, likely hematoma when the hemophilia patient is injured. Its utility, however, extends beyond risk prediction. Because mutant alleles usually constitute sources of malfunctioning protein products, genetic identification of the product can afford access to an otherwise enigmatic etiology. Studies of the Factor VIII allele have facilitated, for example, the determination of the disease's genetic basis, the role of the Factor VIII protein in clotting, and moleular therapeutic options [17].

The strategy of investigating etiology via risk alleles is a legacy of experimental designs that were successfully pursued for the elucidation of biochemical pathways. The presupposition behind these early, now classical approaches conceived of such pathways as linear sequences of progressively altered metabolite products, where each succeeding step entailed a molecular modification and the succession of steps yielded a unique biochemical product. Biochemical pathways fit this decidedly causal and prototypical model. The successive conversion of glucose to pyruvate in the glycolytic pathway, for example, evidenced the stepwise deconstruction by which the larger glucose molecule was gradually disassembled to the smaller pyruvate metabolite. Alleles controlled individual steps through their enzymatic products, which regulated each biochemical change. By rendering the protein products nonfunctional through techniques like mutagenesis given steps of the pathway could be arrested.

Such mutagenesis strategies achieved remarkable success in elucidating pathway steps due to the high specificity and mono-functionality of the enzymes regulating metabolite conversion. Mutation of the gene loci notably yielded focal and highly targeted effects that enabled the reconstruction of the entire pathway, when occurring within a linear sequence and involving a sufficient number of interruptions. By building on naturally occurring lesions, the development of reagents capable of modifying DNA rapidly expanded available tools for DNA dissection. With the advent of molecular biological procedures gene products could be altered at virtually any locus, allowing both pathway reconstruction and characterization of whole clusters of supramolecular assemblies [18].

The success of pathway reconstruction in metabolism led to the implementation of mutagenesis to dissect neural function in simple organisms amenable to genetic manipulation, like *C. elegans* and *Drosophila* on the presupposition that such simple functions were composed of similar molecular sequences; later applied for more complex neural functions like learning. This presupposition was consistent with the nearly universal cellular use of enzymatic catalysis to drive molecular and supramolecular events. It was consistent, moreover, with what was known of causally sequential events that occurred in neural operation, like the activation of synaptic vesicle release following the arrival of an action potential at a synapse. Hence, the use of the strategy extended apparently reasonable presuppositions about the construction of underlying processes to higher neural function.

The success of the mutagenesis strategy for elucidating biochemical pathways, which had motivated its use for exploring neural function, however, was due to a fortuitous confluence that juxtaposed the compositional nature of metabolism - with its linear and precise factory like assembly - with a causal conception involving successive influences effected via steplike sequences. Applied to neural function this conception analogized photopotential generation to a metabolite and the neural events of transduction to successive changes in a single molecular substance. Rather than metering the presence of a physical product, assessments were thus made in terms of the physiological feature, which was viewed as its conceptual equivalent.

Large-scale mutagenesis of fruit flies generated numerous "risk alleles" affecting various components of the photopotential, including its onset, maintenance, termination, and facilitation [19–22]. The strategy usefully characterized highly penetrant alleles with Mendelian-like features, such as those affecting the photopigment protein, and physical components directly mediating the photopotential, like temperature-sensitive channel variants. However, while the strategy yielded numerous novel observations about photoreceptor function—including insight into mechanisms of prolonged potential activation, habituation-like responses, and degenerative cascades—the resolution of transduction per se was less easily and less well resolved. With hindsight and drawing from ongoing parallel studies of phototransduction that did not resort to genetic studies, the lack of resolution may now be partially traced to the conceptual equating of a physical component with a physiological function. Differences in the physical instantiation of a function - as opposed to a metabolite - became notably apparent with the discovery of features such as gated switching, nonlinear dynamical gain and the use of multicomponent protein complexes [23]. For example, generation of the photopotential is critically dependent on the asymmetric distribution of Na and K ions across the photoreceptor cell membrane. Yet, the ionic distribution is not itself generated by the transduction event but is an a priori condition that is required to successfully elicit the photopotential, one that must be maintained continuously against a concentration gradient by energy-consuming ionic pumps. A mutation rendering the pumps ineffective—for example, through a temperature-sensitive, cell mosaic line—would result in the absence of the photopotential and so be interpreted as affecting a step in the transduction pathway. Likewise, the photopotential amplitude displays gain adjustments that enable the detection of intensity variation under widely variant background illumination conditions affecting but not directly constituting the phototransduction events. These observations reveal that unlike the succession of steps occurring in metabolite processing the generation of the photopotential entails a coordinated operation of multiple independent functionalities that are each necessary but not sufficient for the potential to occur. Because each of these functionalities is potentially influenced by multiple alleles, the number of alleles affecting the transduction mechanism is likely to be much larger than that needed in a simple sequence of molecular alterations involving a single substance. In other words, the number of risk alleles that could affect the function is likely to be considerably more than the number of processional events needed to yield the function and indeed is likely to multiply that number. The magnitude of this multiplicative effect becomes especially significant when scaled for complex neural events. Accordingly, differences between the physical mechanisms of metabolism and those of photopotential generation require that the equating of neural function with metabolite processing be reconceived, a conceptual adjustment revealed through the findings of the mutagenesis approach.

3. Massive allelic effects in cognition

Phototransduction clearly constitutes a moderately complex but nonetheless basic function that has evolved to capture light information, in which multiple functionalities work together to yield the photopotential. As a neural mechanism, however, its level of complexity is arguably much less than many behavioral mechanisms operating at systemic and global scales. Motor execution and action identification, for example, require the involvement of visual pathways, task positive frontoparietal networks, premotor and motor cortices, and cerebellar circuits [24]. These are further complicated by the need to evoke egocentric frameworks in goal-directed actions. Consistent with these broad operational requirements, key risk alleles for major cognitive etiopathologies like schizophrenia—with a prevalence of 0.5–1%—are now known to include more than 120 significant loci, that is, alleles that introduce statistically significant changes in manifest clinical symptoms [25]. Moreover, the rate of increase in their discovery has accelerated in recent years, not slowed. Classically, traits governed by large numbers of alleles yield only marginal and quantitative trait variation, with significant changes observed only in cases of rare alleles with high penetrance. Accordingly, many more difficult to detect alleles are likely to also contribute to the manifestation of the disease. In like manner, genetic studies of AD have also identified numerous risk alleles contributing to its etiopathology [26].

Together, the genetic studies show that cognitive diseases, as a group, are polygenic, often influencing hundreds of known alleles with perhaps a much greater unidentified number also influencing disease severity. Variation in behavioral effects due to any single allele, moreover, is small, with observed changes likely to be of a quantitative rather than a qualitative nature. Alone, the use of risk alleles as a strategical undertaking is therefore unlikely to offer significant insight into a causal etiology. The studies, rather, implicate large numbers of affected neurons and circuits, that is, effects likely to be mediated at systemic and even organismal levels of neural function. The range of investigations that have been undertaken over decades of exploration, in fact, from single allele variation to genome-wide investigations reveal that while genetic influences are clearly at work in cognition—such diseases typically display statistically significant familial effects—such influences are apparently mediated through a complex overarching matrix of constraints, one that bears little resemblance to a stepwise biochemical sequence, for which allele study and mutational analyses were first and successfully used.

4. Exploring strategic options in hierarchy

The massive number of affected alleles and the generally enigmatic character of cognitive diseases—more than 13 different, major hypotheses have been advanced to date to explain AD etiopathology—pose significant quandaries in the selection of research strategies, which clearly have as their ultimate objective whole rather than partial and ineffective therapeutic intervention. In light of these realities that seem linked to the extraordinarily complex scales of cognitive operation, the observations from mutagenesis strategies of intermediate-level phenomena like the photopotential offer a strong stimulus for moving beyond purely reductive options in the strategic analysis of cognitive disease etiology.

The recognition that functions often require supramolecular structures, for instance, has motivated the use of proteomics to characterize large-scale protein aggregates. This move would dispense with the lower-level allele studies and focus on how function emerges from clusters of interacting units. Such an approach also holds a promise for its access to the technical virtuosity acquired over decades in the use of translational technologies and analytical protein and peptide biochemistries. In principal virtually any protein segment can now be modified and analyzed to ascertain how such changes causally interact with other protein components to yield specific functions.

For example, the flagellar motor that propels bacterial motion is a well-characterized example of a large supramolecular aggregate consisting of more than seven distinct proteins activated during chemotaxis. Ligand-based stimuli, internal-based phosphorylation modifications, and enhanced protein-binding interactions are now all known events discerned through proteomic studies. These mechanical features are an important aspect of explaining the causal succession for the motor's function, identified in philosophy of science accounts as the "how" question in functional explanation [27]. The motor's performance, however, must also conform to an organizational, that is, design, principle to be functional, which is to say that the explanation for the motor's function must include a dimension beyond that of the succession of internal events leading to functional output. This latter explanation, termed the "why" question, is significant for revealing that efficient causal interactions require the design principle as an a priori condition for their realization, hence, answers to the 'how' question represent only causal outcomes of organizational form.

This invocaton of design principle is significant for identifying the primary causal origin of a function. Rather than determined from below, the mechanistic steps emerge from a predetermined order that is critical for defining material composition and operation. Moreover, the elicited function—the motor's operation, for example—is framed within the context of global organismal need. Accordingly, the emergence of the function is fundamentally related to non-reductive, top-down effects that reflect two aspects of organismal operation; first, an organizational order that governs associations of larger-order complexes (e.g., evident in motifs and network analysis) and, second, a global requirement to satisfy organismal need, seen, for instance, in goal directed activity.

Conceiving of neural function from this higher-order perspective—i.e, dynamically oriented and not static as in the conception of metabolites—has implications for considering the primacy of causes eliciting neural organization—not chiefly through the structuring of its anatomical features, where it is built from the bottom up, but as a dynamic and functional order that has a purposeful orientation, which is determined from the top down.

5. Pursuing top-down strategy in autonomy and goal-directed behavior

Viewed from the dynamic aspect of function, the order of causal priority is reversed where the chief influences underlying organization and performance are systemic and teleological. Lesions of higher-order neural functions, like memory, appear thereby as dysfunctional properties of global representations. Risk alleles, in this reading, and similar reductive approaches can be expected to offer little insight into cognitive operation at the level of neural constructs likely to be impaired in cognitive diseases. Investigations into cognition, instead, seem better directed when exploring the operation of extended networks that function as components of larger systemic or even global operations. By extension, lesions that may fruitfully reveal aspects of large-scale operation are more likely to involve systemic effects that are more closely apposed to global processes mediating organismal tasking.

Models that define the source of this tasking, accordingly, are likely to be helpful for identifying the sorts of lesions that can be usefully exploited for cognitive study. Key features underwriting global cognition notably include those preserving existential independence and the integration of the organism as a whole, that is, those providing for autonomous existence [28]. Understood as a capacity, autonomy implicates dispositional qualities of self-recognition and self-directedness; that is, it invokes self-constructs that elicit higher order operations, which, accordingly, can be disrupted by cognitive disease. As one such higher order operation, for instance, memory is directly elicited by such self constructs in order to facilitate autonomy. Lesions of higher-order capacities like memory, which are evoked by global constructs, may thus be usefully exploited for their properties and manner of elicitation [29, 30].

Emerging from the global operation of the brain, constructs like the self are clearly extraordinarily complex and in many respects seem less tangible than material constituents of reductive and low-level functions. Nonetheless, their organismal reality is clearly evident in manifestations of behavioral activity. For example, the association between a representation of the whole individual by his body and its physical realization in the neural activity of the brain, that is, as a global brain state, is consistently observed in varied perceptual realizations of the self. And in another example the failure of infants in the A not B task to move toward a goal where last seen is interpreted as a failure in motor planning due to maturational insufficiency in mechanisms needed to situate the motor plan that are associated with representing the self as the whole body [31]. These examples suggest that top down aproaches can offer strategic alternatives that more readily yield insight into global brain operations that are manifested at organismal scales.

Indeed, the modern concept of the neural representation of the self, for example, evoked in circumstances where the body is dynamically engaged in intentional actions, is an increasingly well-understood global operation that has emerged from several experimental legacies traced to the notion of the motor image [24]. The image is now known to involve a covert action undertaken only mentally and as a simulation of a non-executed action, with current evidence suggesting that there is a close correspondence between goal-directed information and self-representation [32]. Mechanisms that are likely to shape self-content can therefore be expected to include, for example, cells, circuits, or processes that bear desires and intentions of the author, which are likely to be contained in egocentric networks [33], and which encode agent specific content about an experience. These have been sited to specific domains of the hippocampus, such as the lateral entorhinal cortex where they appear to be influenced by memory recall [34] such as the lateral entorhinal cortex, and to the angular gyrus of the parietal cortex, a region that has been previously identified with self- and bodily representation. Indeed, goal-directed information contained in these networks can be expected to uniquely modify the self-representation by relating the individual to an intended terminus via information that is goal specific.

6. Reconsidering lesions: AD and KS in top-down strategic analysis

The promise of top-down analysis predicts that global organization is selectively impaired at intermediate and even higher levels of brain function, such as those now being investigated through the motor plan. Indeed, disturbances in the sense of self that mark schizophrenia, for example, in prodromal and acute stages, have led to the recognition of the loss of self as a core symptom [35] where both body ownershipa nd sense of agency are impacted [36]. Current evidence on how representational content of the self may be affected and how this may be linked to the body suggest, in fact, that it is mediated through the motor plan, which thereby offers a strategic investigative tool. Insight into the neural features that these results may implicate, for example, can be inferred from misattribution errors that are experimentally evoked in normal individuals and that appear to be pathologically exacerbated in schizophrenic individuals [37].

By extension, memory losses in AD and KS are in their broad features consistent with functional losses that have organismal bearing and that can be revealed through such top-down analysis. Accordingly, this volume represents an effort to forward an argument for global strategies that can be pursued in cognitive etiopathologies. It is a proposal that emerges from the intractability of reductive study faced with the incredible complexity of operation that is intrinsic to cognition. While lacking in the tangible manifestations that have come to mark genetic and molecular study, the reality of global operation is nonetheless manifestly evident. Moreover, it is a reality for which new investigative tools are emerging from research studies, such as the motor plan. Revelation of distinct functional differences in memory loss in diseases like AD and KS, therefore, can be expected to further options for global, top-down study.

Author details

Denis Larrivee[1,2]

1 Loyola University Chicago, Chicago, USA

2 Mind and Brain Group, University of Navarra Medical School, Pamplona, Spain

*Address all correspondence to: sallar1@aol.com

References

[1] Kahlaoui K et al. Neurobiological and neuroethical perspectives on the contribution of functional neuroimaging to the study of aging in the brain. In: Illes J, Sahakian B, editors. Oxford Handbook of Neuroethics. Oxford: Oxford Press; 2011

[2] Larrivee D. Alzheimer's dementia and global self circuits: A new degenerative model? EC Neurology. 2017;**EC0.01**:30-32

[3] Holger J. Memory loss in Alzheimer's disease. Dialogues in Clinical Neuroscience. 2013;**15**(4):445-454

[4] Gold CA, Budson AE. Memory loss in Alzheimer's disease: Implications for development of therapeutics. Expert Review Neurotherapy. 2008;**8**(12):1879-1891

[5] Hellyer PJ et al. The control of global brain dynamics: Opposing actions of frontoparietal control and default mode networks on attention. Journal of Neuroscience. 2014;**34**(2):451-461

[6] Raichle M. Two views of brain functioning. In: Auletta G, Colage I, Jeannerod M, editors. Brains Top Down: Is Top-Down Causation Challenging Neuroscience? London: World Scientific; 2013

[7] Zhong Y et al. Altered effective connectivity patterns of the default mode network in Alzheimer's disease: An fMRI study. Neuroscience Letters. 2014;**578**:171-175

[8] Cordova-Palomera A et al. Disrupted global metastability and static and dynamic brain connectivity across individuals in the Alzheimer's disease continuum. Scientific Reports. 2017;**7**(40268):1-6

[9] Arts NJM, Walvoort SJW, Kessels RPC. Korsakoff's syndrome. Neuropsychiatric Disease and Treatment. 2017;**13**:2875-2890

[10] Markowitsch HJ. Memory and self-neuroscientific landscapes. ISRN Neuroscience. 2013;**2013**:1-26

[11] Kessels RPC, Kopelman MD. Context memory in Korsakoff's syndrome. Neuropsychology Review. 2012;**22**:117-131

[12] Gibson GE, Hirsch JA, et al. Vitamin B1 (thiamine) and dementia. Annals of the New York Academy of Sciences. 2016;**1367**(1):21-30

[13] Moss et al. Differential patterns of memory loss among patients with Alzheimer's disease, Huntington's disease, and alcoholic Korsakoff's syndrome. Archives of Neurology. 1986;**43**(3):239-246. DOI: 10.1001/archneur.1986.00520030031008

[14] Oberle I et al. Genetic screening for hemophilia a (classic hemophilia) with a polymorphic DNA probe. New England Journal of Medicine. 1985;**312**:682-686

[15] Schwab SG, Wildenauer DB. Genetics of psychiatric disorders in the GWAS era: An update on schizophrenia. European Archive of Psychiatry and Clinical Neuroscience. 2013;**263**(Suppl 2):S147-S154

[16] Celeste M, Karch A, Goate M. Alzheimer's disease risk genes and mechanisms of disease pathogenesis. Biological Psychiatry. 2015;77(1):43-51

[17] Ringman JM et al. Genetic heterogeneity in Alzheimer disease and implications for treatment strategies. Current Neurology and Neuroscience Report. 2014;**14**:499. DOI: 10.1007/s11910-014-0499-8

[18] Vizcaíno JA et al. A guide to the proteomics identifications database proteomics data repository. Proteomics. 2009;**9**(18):4276-4283

[19] Pak WK, Istrit SE, Deland MC, Wu CF. Photoreceptor mutant of Drosophila: Is a protein involved in intermediate steps of phototransduction. Science. 1976;**194**(4268):956-959

[20] Guan Z, Buhl LK, Quinn WG, Littleton JT. Altered gene regulation and synaptic morphology in Drosophila learning and memory mutants. Learning and Memory. Cold Spring Harbor. 2011;**18**(4):191-206

[21] Pearn MT, Randall LL, Shortridge RD, Burg MG, Pak WL. Molecular, biochemical, and electrophysiological characterization of Drosophila norpA mutants. The Journal of Biological Chemistry. 1996;**271**(9):4937-4945

[22] Papazian DM et al. Cloning of genomic and complementary DNA from Shaker, a putative potassium channel gene. Science. 1987;**237**(4816):749-753

[23] Pepperberg DR. Transduction gain in light adaptation of rod photoreceptors. The Journal of General Physiology. 2001;**117**(4):361-364

[24] Jeannerod M. Levels of representation of goal-directed actions. In: Fruend HJ, Jeannerod M, Hallett M, Leiguarda M, editors. Higher-Order Motor Disorders. Oxford: Oxford University Press; 2005

[25] Ripke et al. Genome-wide association analysis identifies 14 new risk loci for schizophrenia. Nature Genetics. 2013;**45**(10):1150-1159

[26] Guerreiro RJ et al. The genetic architecture of Alzheimer's disease: Beyond APP, PSENs and APOE. Neurobiology of Aging. 2010, 2010;**33**(3):437-456

[27] Braillard PA. Systems biology and the mechanistic framework. History Philosophy Life Science. 2010;**32**(1):43-62

[28] Moreno A, Mossio M. Biological Autonomy: A Philosophical and Theoretical Inquiry. Dordrecht: Springer Publishing; 2015

[29] Ruiz-Mirazo K, Moreno A. Autonomy in evolution: From minimal to complex life. Synthese. 2012;**185**:21-52

[30] Christensen WD, Bickhard MH. The process dynamics of normative function. The Monist. 2002;**85**:3-28

[31] Smith L. Stability and flexibility in development. In: Spencer J, Thomas MSC, McClelland JL, editors. Toward a Unified Theory of Development. Oxford: Oxford University Press; 2009

[32] Jeannerod M. The sense of agency and its disturbances in schizophrenia: A reappraisal. Experimental Brain Research. 2009;**192**(3):527-532

[33] Wang C, Chen X, Lee H, Deshmukh SS, Yoganarasimha D, et al. Egocentric coding of external items in the lateral entorhinal cortex. Science. 2018;**362**(6417):945-949

[34] Bonini L et al. Grasping neurons of monkey parietal and premotor cortices encode action goals at distinct levels of abstraction during complex action sequences. Neuroscience. 2011;**31**(15):5876-5887

[35] Ferri F, Frassinetti F, Mastrangelo F, Salone A, Ferro FM, et al. Bodily self and schizophrenia: The loss of implicit self-body knowledge. Conscious Cognition. 2012;**21**(3):1365-1374

[36] Aaron F et al. Disrupted modularity and local connectivity of brain functional networks in childhood onset schizophrenia. Frontiers in Systems Neuroscience. 2010;**4**(147):1-16

[37] Van den Bos E, Jeannerod M. Sense of body and sense of action both contribute to self-recognition. Cognition. 2002;**85**:177-187

Section 2

Alzheimers: Enigmatic Conclusions from Science

Chapter 2

Fact, Fiction, or Evolution: Mechanism Hypothesis of Alzheimer's Disease

José V. Pardo

Abstract

The metabolism hypothesis of Alzheimer's disease (AD) was first proposed in 1975. In normal aging and very mild AD, the cerebral metabolic rate for oxygen (CMRO2) and cerebral blood flow (CBF) remained approximately constant, but the metabolism of glucose (CMRglu) declined markedly. This decline in CMRglu identified a specific and primary metabolic defect that triggered downstream cellular cascades evolving into AD and its characteristic neuropathological lesions. These findings led research about AD into the role of insulin resistance that foresaw modern trials of insulin for AD treatment. The metabolism hypothesis evolved over subsequent decades with improved in-vivo measurement of metabolic parameters and AD biomarkers in humans. A more recent model highlights the interrelationships between the default mode network (DMN) and biomarkers such as CMRglu, amyloid, and tau. In other words, metabolic conditions related to sustained cortical activity during aging throughout the lifetime are conducive to the deposition of amyloid. This activity is thought to underlie the "autobiographical self." These ideas and findings motivate aging and AD-research focus on the biochemistry and cell biology of cerebral metabolism.

Keywords: dementia, amyloid, tau, cerebral metabolism, default mode networks, cerebral energetics, aerobic glycolysis, cognitive aging, functional connectivity

1. Introduction

Hoyer et al. proposed the metabolism hypothesis of AD based on observations of normal aging and early AD focusing on the relationships between CMRglu, CMRO, and CBF [1–3]. This hypothesis has both weak and strong versions. The weak version, not of interest here, suggests that amyloid deposition is an epiphenomenon, potentially unrelated to AD; the causative pathophysiology must lay elsewhere—perhaps a primary mitochondrial failure. The more interesting hypothesis relies on a stronger version: neural activity sustained during resting and introspection (i.e., wakefulness [4]) over a lifetime (i.e., the "autobiographical self") drives AD pathology.

A more recent model of the strong version posited sustained metabolic activity in the default mode network (DMN) is a substrate for amyloid deposition through the mediation of some process related to neural activity [5]. CMRglu declined with aging. Since oxidative metabolism was largely preserved, a primary abnormality in

IntechOpen

the handling of glucose was posited with the observation that aerobic glycolysis (AG) declined precipitously during normal aging [6, 7]. Concomitantly, molecular imaging of critical biomarkers in AD identified for the first time the distribution of proteins such as fibrillar amyloid and tau in the brain, both in asymptomatic healthy elderly and in patients with various neurodegenerative disorders including AD [8–10].

Such progress led to the definition and characterization of preclinical and clinical AD based on biomarkers for staging [11–14]. To understand the pathophysiology of the hypothesized metabolic dysfunction, understanding the relationships between brain metabolism and these neuropathological biomarkers became critical during both normal aging and AD. These advances detail the evolution of imaging biomarkers along with their relationship to the brain's structural, metabolic, and cognitive dysfunction.

Here, recent findings relevant to aging and AD are reviewed briefly as background. Current understanding of the development and ontogenesis of biomarkers for AD are summarized. Data are integrated with advances in neuroimaging and brain metabolism as well as in preclinical models mostly focusing on the resting state. These results bear on the metabolism hypothesis of AD. Notable gaps in this hypothesis and its relationship to cognitive aging highlight avenues requiring further research for progress in the field.

2. Amyloid and tau in aging and AD

Several studies of patients developing dementia (both early and late-onset sporadic AD; familial AD) as well as Down's syndrome show amyloid deposition begins decades before overt symptoms of dementia arise [11, 15, 16]. Amyloid deposition of plaques, particularly the diffuse type, in AD begins in inferior neocortex with spread to other neocortical regions including precuneus, lateral parietal, and frontal association neocortices [17, 18]. Amyloid positivity predicts past and future progressive cognitive decline [19]. Glucose metabolism tends to decline where amyloid localizes; it is first seen in preclinical AD, mild cognitive impairment (MCI), and early AD using fluorodeoxyglucose (FDG) positron emission tomography (PET) in the posterior cingulate cortex (PCC) followed by biparietal involvement [20–22]. The steepest increases in amyloid deposition during healthy aging according to amyloid PET, thought to measure fibrillar amyloid or neuritic plaques, occurs in anterior cingulate cortex (ACC), PCC, precuneus, and temporal cortices [23]. The earliest detectable amyloid deposits by PET localize to precuneus, PCC, and medial orbitofrontal cortex; these deposits were not associated with atrophy or hypometabolism despite changes in functional connectivity [24].

Although there is some overlap between amyloid deposition and cortical hypometabolism [22], other factors such as APOE genotype and tau deposition affect the distribution of amyloid. Whole-brain amyloid positivity appears a greater determinant of gross cognitive dysfunction compared to the precise areal distribution; however, measures of non-crystallized intelligence (e.g., executive functions, reasoning, problem solving) are sensitive to the amount deposited [19]. It is not unusual to find a dissociation between amyloid deposition and metabolic hypometabolism or between amyloid deposition and cortical thinning [25–27]. As discussed below (Section 6.1), while clinically normal elders can show significant correlation between thinning and amyloid deposition in the PCC, they do not show a significant association between these biomarkers in the ACC [28]. Amyloid deposition although predictive of future cognitive decline correlates poorly with actual cognitive status: the number of neurofibrillary tangles (NFTs), not senile amyloid plaques, correlates with cognitive status before death [29]. Classically, amyloid is necessary but not sufficient for the diagnosis of AD; tau with neurofibrillary changes is also required [30, 31]. However, over one-third of patients with clinically diagnosed mild to moderate AD who do not carry an APOE4 allele show minimal amyloid yet extensive neurofibrillary degeneration on autopsy [32]. Whether this group is pathophysiologically an AD variant or a tauopathy remains unclear [32, 33].

Deposits of tau generally follow amyloid. Immunohistochemical studies of tau and neuroimaging of humans using tau radiotracers converge on tau's more restricted involvement in the temporal lobe in early AD [17, 34, 35]. Tau does not follow the global miliary pattern of amyloid neocortical involvement with disease progression. Tau's presence more directly correlates with cognitive dysfunction and cortical thinning than does amyloid [14, 36]. These changes reflect presumably the final stages of neurodegeneration. Unlike amyloid deposition, the localization of tau mirrors the clinical and neuroanatomical phenotypic variability of AD [37, 38]. Longitudinal data of both amyloid and tau have enabled assessment of directionality of biomarker spread as well as potential relationships with gene expression [39]. APOE played a central role in the lipid interactome affecting both Aß and tau spread, while tau- and Aß-risk genes differentially contributed to the specific spread of each biomarker.

3. The default mode network (DMN)

The distribution of amyloid has been noted to overlap with the neural system related to the default mode of brain function [5]. The observation has prompted hypotheses about the relationship of neural activity, the default mode network, and AD that continue to evolve.

PET studies have shown a broad region of relative deactivation in resting states compared to active states with greatest deactivation within the ventromedial prefrontal cortex (VMPFC) with peak minimum at Brodmann area 10 (BA10; **Figure 1**) [40]. Additional regions showing deactivations localized bilaterally to the inferior and superior frontal cortex, PCC/precuneus, prefrontal cortex, inferior parietal cortex, and several temporal areas.

The deactivation in the VMPFC during rest was shown not to reflect a relative activation as the OEF did not change significantly from whole-brain (e.g., **Figure 1**;

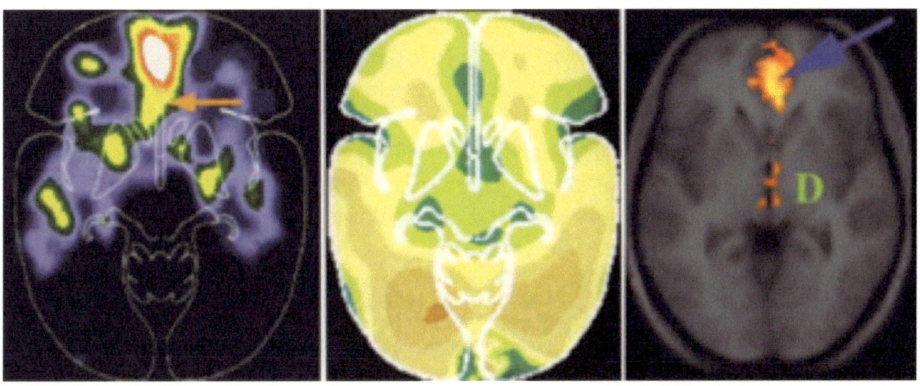

Figure 1.
Transverse sections (z = −6) of stereotactically normalized parametric data showing convergence across studies between CBF change and FC as well as relative stability of OEF. Left: Region of common relative CBF deactivation (VMPFC) in mega image contrast between active scans and passive scans (peak Z-score − 7.7; modified from [40]); middle: Default mode oxygen extraction fraction during rest with eyes closed; uniform OEF; no OEF increase in VMPFC [41]. Right: Resting state FC of the VMPFC with the DMN [49]. Middle & left: Copyright (2003) National Academy of Sciences, U.S.A.

Raichle et al. [41]). If the VMPFC were activated, it should show increased OEF (as some regions in the visual cortices, see red color). The activated network during passive tasks was hypothesized instead to reflect a return to baseline or default mode network (DMN) that was interrupted by active tasks. The regional specificity of the DMN suggested some ill-defined brain function.

The DMN can be detected even in the presence of deep anesthesia suggesting a degree of invariance with respect to consciousness possibly reflecting intrinsic brain organization such as anatomical connectivity [42]. The VMPFC becomes more active not only at rest relative to other active task states (e.g., attentional) but also during a variety of other conditions where attention is directed away from the external environment. Such states include introspection, "mind wandering" [43], self-appraisal or introspection [44], stimulus independent thought [45], episodic future simulation, trait emotional self-awareness [46], and interoceptive tasks (e.g., recall of visceral information) [47]. As this book notes, these are reflections of the "autobiographical self."

Previous work in the mid to late 1990s observed physiological fluctuations occurring during active states and even during rest in the MR blood oxygen level dependent (BOLD) signal in humans and in CBF in rodents that were correlated at low frequency (0.1 Hz) across regions known to have anatomical and functional relatedness [48]. However, it remained unclear how these temporal signals related to the DMN as defined from PET studies.

Remarkably, when the VMPFC region in the DMN (showing relative deactivation during active tasks using PET) was used as a seed region to correlate BOLD signals throughout the brain, a network surface based on interregional temporal coherence of the BOLD MR signal that was visually superimposable on the DMN. Use of a spiral MR pulse sequence avoiding signal dropout in ventral prefrontal regions enabled good signal recovery within VMPFC (**Figure 1** [49]). Subsequent fMRI studies examining resting state networks displayed a more variable pattern in the medial prefrontal regions frequently showing more dorsal localization [50–52]. The significance of this disparity is unclear but may relate to low signal recovery with fMRI in ventral brain regions or other subnetworks (see below).

The analysis of BOLD data from the resting state using independent component analysis of FC identified numerous subnetworks showing both anatomical (known afferent and efferent anatomical projections) and functional (coactivation during tasks) architecture converging with other datasets (**Figure 2**) [53]. The four principal RSNs are the dorsal attention network (DAN), DMN (as above), salience network (SAL; also termed cingulo-opercular), and bilateral frontoparietal control network (FPC). The latter is sometimes segmented to dorsal and ventral systems [54].

The precise components of these RSNs need further refinement. For example, how does the "anterior medial prefrontal cortex" relate to VMPFC, pgACC, dACC, and medial superior frontal gyrus? What elementary cognitive operations do these different areas serve? Similarly, how does the "PCC/precuneus" relate to the various medial parietal subregions, and what functions do they serve? In this regard, preliminary dissection divides the PCC into dorsal and ventral regions, each with two additional subregions that in turn connect with other differing cortical projection regions [55].

These four major networks based on data averaged across individuals only hint at the complexity on a more fine-grained analysis. ICA can produce many more networks, and the Human Connectome Project points to 180 parcels per hemisphere [56]. When resting BOLD is collected over many hours for one individual, much more complex, interdigitated, parallel, distributed networks become apparent without the blurring caused by inter-subject averaging [57].

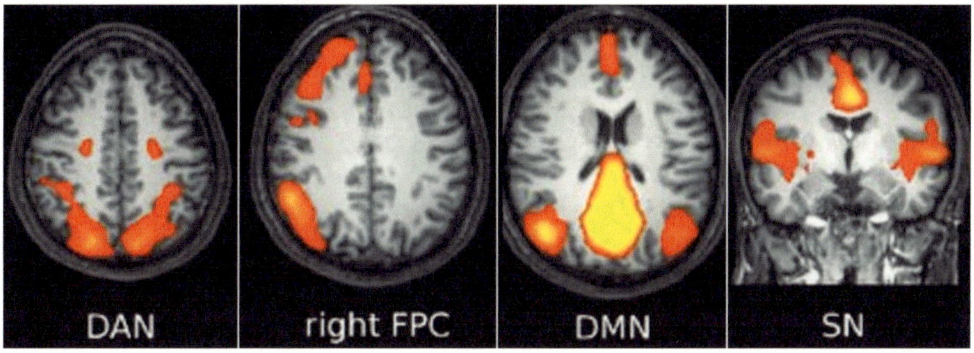

Figure 2.
Four major RSNs revealed by ICA: DAN, dorsal attention network; DMN, default mode network; SN, salience network (also called cingulo-opercular network); right FPC, frontoparietal control network. Modified from [54].

Data on the effects of aging and amyloid/tau deposition on these subnetworks continue to accrue, but there appears differential vulnerability of different subnetworks. For example, amyloid decreased the FC of the DMN subnetworks relevant to episodic memory (PCC, angular gyrus, VMPFC) while increasing FC in dorsolateral and anterior medial prefrontal cortices as well as lateral temporal regions [58]. The latter regions were interpreted as reflecting compensatory responses to the amyloid-related dysfunction in the memory subnetworks. Furthermore, the mere presence of biomarkers such as amyloid in preclinical AD can confound FC findings within and across RSNs. Cognitively normal subjects without vs. with amyloid positivity show small vs. large age-related changes in RSN functional, respectively [59].

The DMN shares considerable connectivity with the hippocampus [60, 61]. The DMN couples with different sectors of the hippocampus [62] through the parahippocampal gyrus depending on task context during rest [63]; spontaneous, unconstrained thought (e.g., thinking about one's past or future [64]); episodic memory retrieval [65]; and associative episodic memory encoding [63]. This network becomes disrupted early occurring both in preclinical and early AD (see Section 6, below) [60, 66].

4. Cerebral energetics

The energetic balance sheet indicates a large part of oxidative metabolism maintains the resting state [67–69]. The classic work of Seymour Kety showed oxygen consumption in the brain differed little across a wide variety of abnormal mental states such as in psychosis, whether in schizophrenic decompensation or acute drug intoxication [70]. In response to external stimulation, the brain only increases oxygen consumption by 5% [71]. Similarly, few differences in oxygen consumption occur between sleep vs. wakefulness [72]. Although the bulk of brain work at rest and on activation derives from oxidative phosphorylation [71], the metabolism hypothesis of AD focuses on a specific metabolic pathway: AG (i.e., glycolysis in the presence of adequate levels of oxygen; i.e., nonoxidative metabolism of glucose [73]).

Regions high in oxidative phosphorylation do not necessarily have high rates of AG. As an example, the visual cortex has very high glucose metabolism; high cerebral blood flow (CBF); high oxidative metabolism (cerebral metabolic rate for oxygen) with high levels of cytochrome oxidase; but low AG [73]. The focus on AG follows from the visual cortex having relative resistance to amyloid deposition and being one of the regions showing little decrease in metabolism with aging. In contrast, the PCC has high flow, oxidative metabolism, glucose metabolism, and high

AG [73]. As summarized above, the PCC is very susceptible to amyloid deposition and is among the earliest dysfunctional regions in AD. These observations further refined the metabolism hypothesis of AD.

In a group of mostly cognitively intact elders, those globally without amyloid did not have tau accumulation in areas prone toward tau deposits (precuneus, amygdala, entorhinal, inferior temporal, inferior and superior parietal, fusiform, and lateral occipital cortices) and did not have decreased CMRO or AG [69]. They showed a positive correlation between AG and CMRglu; no correlations surfaced between CMRO, CMRglu, or tau deposition. In contrast, those who were amyloid positive globally showed an inverse relationship between tau and AG but not between tau and CMRO or CMRglu. These data suggest the loss of AG in tau-prone regions with tau accumulation leads to decreased plasticity and decreased neuroprotection (i.e., decreased redox buffering) leading to accelerated tauopathy.

5. Role of DMN and amyloid

The default network shows overlap with brain regions high in AG which in turn show overlap with areas of amyloid deposition in AD [74]. Unlike oxidative phosphorylation used to generate energy, AG proceeds less efficiently energetically (2 ATP vs. 38 ATP per glucose molecule) but more suitably for reduction of biomolecules for anabolism [75]. Anabolism that appears to play a much greater role in early human development could also provide, albeit to a lesser extent, the substrates for plasticity related to learning and memory in adults [76, 77]. The metabolism hypothesis is important because it motivates the search for AD pathophysiology beyond amyloid deposition to some aspect of cerebral metabolism particularly AG. Normal aging is associated with the loss of AG in regions which sustain higher levels of AG in youth; these are the very regions showing susceptibility to amyloid deposition [7]. The metabolism hypothesis could help explain why the frequency of AD rises relentlessly with aging and oxidative stress.

Several lines of evidence support the metabolism hypothesis of AD through altered processing of Aß [78]. The processing pathways include both increased production and decreased clearance. Most AD-causing dominant mutations in APP, PSEN1, and PSEN2 increase Aß production [79]. One mutation that is protective for AD occurs near the APP BACE1 cleavage site impairing γ cleavage; it is associated in vitro with decreased amyloidogenic peptides [80]. Likewise, vibrissal stimulation of APP transgenic mice increases Aß in interstitial CSF and amyloid plaques while decreasing lactate, a proxy for neural activity [81]. In-vitro mouse slice preparations show based on microdialysis rapid increases in Aß correlated with synaptic activity [82]. In cognitively normal older adults, greater hippocampal activity during encoding at baseline correlates with longitudinal amyloid deposition and diminished cognitive performance [83]. APOE, the major risk locus for AD, plays a key role in Aß aggregation, fibrillogenesis, and maturation of neuritic plaques [84]. AD patients relative to controls have decreased clearance of CSF Aß with normal rate of Aß production [85].

6. Gaps in the metabolism hypothesis

Here, issues informing discussions about the amyloid hypothesis of AD and relationships to cerebral metabolism are outlined. These raise questions about the strong version of the metabolism hypothesis and its implications, or at least suggest a need for revision. Significant circumstantial evidence centers on several observations: (1) normal cognitive aging; (2) familial AD; (3) healthy individuals at very high risk of AD (*APOE*E4* homozygotes); (4) the evolving role of tau in AD; (5) interrelationships between amyloid and tau in AD pathology; and (6) the implications for cognitive function in "real time."

6.1 The metabolism hypothesis and cognitive aging

The metabolism hypothesis suggests that if chronically elevated levels of resting brain activity over the lifetime drive Aß deposition with attendant cognitive dysfunction leading to AD, there should be amyloid deposition during healthy aging as well. Based on this mechanism, the PCC region should show major hypometabolism, atrophy, and amyloid deposition as seen in early AD [21, 86–88].

Yet, this phenomenon is not observed. The PCC in normal aging shows relative preservation (**Figure 3**). Among the regions showing the least decline in metabolism with aging is the PCC. Older healthy adults show minimal PCC atrophy rates over 12 months [89]. Older healthy adults, especially E4 non-carriers, do not show amyloid deposition in the PCC [90–92]. Young adult E4 carriers with positive family history of AD and at high risk of future AD already show PCC hypometabolism implying DMN hyperactivity related to AD must have occurred before then [93]. Of note, older healthy E4 non-carriers begin to show amyloid positivity at around 71 years of age, while the E4 carriers develop amyloid positivity about 20 years earlier. Interestingly, when separating the independent effects of aging vs. E4 load, amyloid deposition shows a more frontal involvement. Of note, the effects of aging and E4 load interact: the peak hazard ratio occurs ~60 years of age and declines thereafter; E4 is a risk factor for AD even for younger adults (<65 years) [94]. Furthermore, resting connectivity of the PCC/precuneus region to the ACC is reduced in older healthy adults who carry E4 even in the absence of detectable fibrillar amyloid or decreased CSF Aß42 suggesting both Aß-dependent and Aß-independent aging-related mechanisms [95].

The principal locus of declining metabolism in healthy elders does not map to the PCC but localizes instead to the ACC (**Figure 3**) [96–101]. ACC hypometabolism correlates also with aging-related decline in cognitive function [99]. Whereas

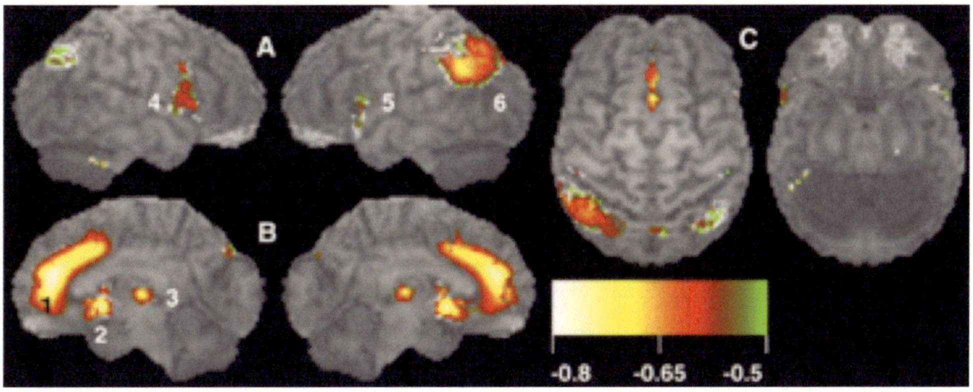

Figure 3.
Decline of brain activity with aging in healthy volunteers. Voxel-wise Pearson correlation (r) map of glucose uptake vs. age in stereotactically normalized brain (3D-SSP; S. Minoshima, University of Utah). A, lateral; B, medial; C, dorsal (left)/ventral (right). Color scale shows peak r = −0.8. Note the greatest decline in glucose uptake with age localizes to the ACC (BA 32/9; region 1). A midline circuit (regions 1-3) includes dorsomedial thalamus and basal forebrain/subgenual cingulate; the metabolism in this circuit correlates with declining executive function (verbal fluency). Other regions with lower correlations are not associated with cognitive performance. Reprinted from Neuroimage, Vol 35(3), Pardo JV et al., Where the brain grows old: Decline in anterior cingulate and medial prefrontal function with normal aging. Copyright (2007), with permission from Elsevier.

AG localizes to ACC, PCC, and parietal regions, loss of regions high in AG during youth appears to occur in all three regions without selectivity for any one of these regions [76]. So, unless AD per se involves hyperactivity of the DMN beyond that in normal elders for which there is no evidence, the hypothesis does not address the inconsistency between mechanisms of cognitive aging versus AD to account for the observed dissociation between ACC and PCC findings.

Several observations related to cognitive aging need reconciliation with the metabolism hypothesis. Healthy elders free from amyloid deposition show a remarkable disconnection between the anterior and posterior default networks (i.e., ACC and PCC) [102]. Yet, nothing about the metabolism hypothesis explains why DMN regions with high AG, where amyloid will be deposited as AD develops, should disconnect—both regions should show aging-related hypometabolism as a result of white matter damage. Similarly, cognitively normal elders not at high risk for AD (no E4) show increases and decreases within anterior DMN connectivity, while showing only decreases in posterior DMN FC [103]. Cognitively intact elders with minimal amyloid deposition without E4 have greater connectivity of the ACC to the precuneus than those with E4 [95]. The aging-related anterior vs. posterior dissociations in connectivity within DMN networks remain theoretically difficult to predict based solely on the metabolism hypothesis.

The ACC also has high glucose metabolism, flow, oxygen consumption, and AG; yet, the ACC does not show amyloid deposition akin to the PCC with healthy aging (those >60 years without amyloid positive scans [23]). Thus, chronic neural activity along with AG during the lifespan per se is not sufficient to lay down amyloid. Just as PCC hypometabolism marks focal atrophy early in AD, the region of ACC hypometabolism with aging should likewise display cortical thinning. However, several large studies do not support the prediction [104, 105], although not all findings are convergent [106]. Additionally, recent studies of tau deposition in preclinical AD show early deposition in the PCC but not in the ACC [107]. Those elders with cognitive function akin to much younger subjects (i.e., "SuperAgers") show thickening of the ACC and increased spindle cells suggestive of plasticity with aging; or alternatively, "SuperAgers" may be endowed with ACC thickening before aging [108, 109]. Also, age can confound years of education; the latter is associated with increased ACC thickness and metabolism [110, 111]. However, studies of the effects of aerobic fitness exercise on cognition and cortex show ACC thickening in older adults in support of the potential for plasticity in this region [112].

A clear dissociation can arise also between amyloid deposition and FDG metabolism in the ACC in AD that is difficult to explain with the metabolism hypothesis. Patients who initially had mild AD, as confirmed with metabolic and amyloid biomarkers, were followed for 2 years along with a matched, amyloid negative control group. Despite extensive amyloid deposition in the ACC of the AD patients, no hypometabolism colocalized in the ACC during follow-up [22]. The aging-related ACC hypometabolism noted previously likely led to a floor effect across groups. Likewise, aging-related ACC hypometabolism would tend to spare amyloid deposition in patients appearing inconsistent with the metabolism hypothesis given extensive amyloid involvement of the ACC in AD.

6.2 The metabolism hypothesis and autosomal dominant AD

A corollary of the metabolism hypothesis suggests those with familial AD would show similar patterns of hypometabolism and amyloid deposition to late-onset, sporadic AD. However, those with mutations (APP, PSEN1, PSEN2) show greatest amyloid deposition in the basal ganglia, a site that only becomes involved late in typical sporadic AD [113–115]. However, the specific pattern of amyloid deposition may depend to some extent on the specific mutation. For example, the PS1 mutation, E280A, shows amyloid deposition more like late-onset sporadic AD than many other mutations with early onset. This variability may not surprise given the complexity of the underlying biology of different mutations in PS1 [116].

6.3 Role of APOE genotype in the metabolism hypothesis

If regional brain activity drives amyloid deposition in the pattern seen in AD, then the AD metabolic pattern should arise in those at highest risk for the future development of AD—asymptomatic *APOE*E4* homozygotes, who have a 12-fold increased risk of LOAD. So far, there are seven such individuals in the Alzheimer's Disease Neuroimaging Initiative's (ADNI) database. Their pattern of amyloid deposition highlights bilateral lenticular nuclei and the ACC/medial prefrontal involvement with the PCC notably unaffected (see **Figure 3**). In fact, the deposition of amyloid in the homozygotes is reminiscent of that seen in Down's syndrome and most mutations found in autosomal dominantly inherited forms of AD arising in APP, PS1, or PS2 [113–115, 117]. This pattern of amyloid deposition in E4 homozygotes is consistent with findings reported previously in an independent group of eight homozygotes [91].

6.4 Role of tau in the metabolism hypothesis

Another difficulty with the metabolism hypothesis of AD is the notable absence of tau involvement in this theory. The role of tau, its modifications, and its etiologic role in neurodegeneration in AD has been reviewed previously [118]. Although the metabolism hypothesis of AD focuses on amyloid deposition, there is increasing evidence that tau plays at least as great if not greater etiopathological role. Of interest in this context, recent studies show tau deposition during preclinical AD in the PCC; the metabolism hypothesis cannot explain this dissociation between PCC and ACC [107].

AD cases with neurofibrillary changes (neuritic plaques, neurofibrillary tangles, neurofibrillary threads, tau tangles) typically show extensive amyloid deposition. However, not all cases with extensive amyloid deposition show neurofibrillary changes [17]. Amyloid deposits and neuritic plaques vary widely across individuals both temporally and regionally; so, they do not provide useful biomarkers for staging of AD [17]. In contrast, the distribution of tau is consistent across individuals and provides useful staging of disease progression [17].

Hyper-phosphorylated intraneuronal tau ("pretangle") has been reported even in young adults in the absence of amyloid particularly in subcortical nuclei such as the locus coeruleus [119]. The significance of these findings in the context of AD remains uncertain as the pretangle material may be transient, related incidentally to other processes (e.g., traumatic brain injury), or the earliest manifestations of AD. Furthermore, studies of transgenic mice with APOE isoform knock-in and APOE knock-out show that even in the absence of amyloid, E4 is particularly neurotoxic in mice with mutant tau transgenes, and this toxicity is in part mediated by neuroinflammation via the innate immune system produced by microglia and type A1 astrocytes [120].

A recent study identified the significant role of tau in the context of amyloid deposition [121]. High resolution fMRI of cerebral blood volume (CBV), coupled to regional metabolism, mapped the earliest changes in preclinical AD to lateral entorhinal (LEC), transentorhinal, and perirhinal cortices, as predicted from neuropathological studies [17]. The former region's CBV correlated significantly with a test of delayed retention. Three lines of mice were generated with differential expression in entorhinal cortex of pathological human APP, tau, or both transgenes.

Mice with mutant entorhinal tau alone, but not mutant APP alone, had diminished CBV in LEC with aging [121]. The double mutant had decreased LEC CBV with aging compared to the single mutants and other controls thereby demonstrating that APP increased tau-related metabolic dysfunction. Decreased CBV in aged double mutant spread even to posterior parietal cortex, a pattern reminiscent of human AD. APP immunohistochemistry of older mice showed no changes between mutant APP and double mutant mice; the label localized mostly to entorhinal cortex. However, tau immunohistochemistry of older mice showed increased signal in the double mutants with the suggestion of relocalization of phospho-tau from neuropil to the somatodendritic compartment.

The differing roles of amyloid and tau in the evolution of AD were recently highlighted in cognitively intact elders [58]. Those positive for amyloid (Aß+) showed hyperconnectivity within DMN and SN when tau deposits were low. In contrast, the Aß + subjects showed decreased FC with increasing tau deposition. Thus, the effects of PET biomarkers on FC appear complex and likely involve multiple neuropathological processes.

These data make clear that tau cannot be ignored in understanding the ontogenesis of AD. The metabolism hypothesis needs modification for relevance beyond amyloid deposition to AD pathophysiology.

6.5 Cognitive processing in "real time"

The biomarkers discussed so far are not dynamic in terms of real time. These scans, even when measured during rest, probe parameters over many minutes—totally divorced from cognitive processes that occur at the scale of milliseconds to seconds. Recent studies hint that the metabolism hypothesis has relevance to the latter time scale.

As mentioned in Section 5, lactate is a proxy for neural activation and through regulation of $NADH/NAD^+$ becomes a modulator of rCBF in response to activation [122]. Astrocytes on activation show a metabolic switch toward AG shifting oxygenation from astrocytes to neurons [123]. In turn, lactate produced through AG is critical for memory formation [124]. Because AG can provide reducing equivalents for biosynthesis of macromolecules for plasticity, learning tasks demonstrate focal increases in AG on-line with experience-dependent plasticity [77]. The elevation in AG can persist for many minutes after an activation task [125]. How amyloid impacts real-time learning through changes in AG remains to be elucidated.

Preliminary studies have examined using magnetoencephalography (MEG) oscillatory power in real time in cognitively normal elders either with amyloid deposition ("preclinical AD") or without amyloid deposition [126]. Increases in power in the alpha range in the amyloid-positive preclinical cases at rest localized over the ACC and correlated with increased glucose metabolism. These metabolic changes did not yet correlate with structural atrophy or cognitive decline. The findings begin to define the earliest on-line physiological changes in preclinical AD. Similarly, increased functional connectivity at rest localized to the ACC. Proposed hypotheses include cognitive compensation (i.e., cognitive reserve) or amyloid-related hyper-excitability in preclinical AD [58, 127].

7. Concluding remarks about the metabolism hypothesis

The observations reviewed above argue that even if chronic neural activity in the DMN biases Aß production and clearance toward amyloid deposition, different mechanisms participate in Aß localization in normal elderly, E4 homozygotes, familial dominant AD, and sporadic AD. Further, tau has reached a new level of significance in AD pathophysiology. The cellular and molecular mechanisms of human Aß deposition and the relationship to AD appear pleiomorphic and complex defy so far simplistic explanations for a complex disease. However, given the recent advances in multimodal molecular imaging (amyloid, tau, neuroinflammation, etc.), the story is likely to evolve quickly.

Acknowledgements

This work was supported by the Minneapolis Veterans Health Care System; the University of Minnesota Libraries Open Access Fund; and Merit Award I01CX000501 (VA CSR&D).

Conflict of interest

The author declares no conflict of interest.

Author details

José V. Pardo[1,2]

1 Department of Psychiatry, University of Minnesota, Minneapolis, USA

2 Cognitive Neuroimaging Unit, Mental Health Service Line, Minneapolis Veterans Health Care System, Minneapolis, USA

*Address all correspondence to: jvpardo@umn.edu

References

[1] Hoyer S. The abnormally aged brain. Its blood flow and oxidative metabolism. A review—Part II. Archives of Gerontology and Geriatrics. 1982;**1**(3):195-207

[2] Hoyer S. The young-adult and normally aged brain. Its blood flow and oxidative metabolism. A review—Part I. Archives of Gerontology and Geriatrics. 1982;**1**(2):101-116

[3] Hoyer S, Oesterreich K, Weinhardt F, Kruger G. Blood flow and oxidative metabolism of the brain in patients with dementia (author's transl). Journal of Neurology. 1975;**210**(4):227-237

[4] Kang J-E, Lim MM, Bateman RJ, Lee JJ, Smyth LP, Cirrito JR, et al. Amyloid-β dynamics are regulated by orexin and the sleep-wake cycle. Science. 2009;**326**(5955):1005-1007

[5] Buckner R, Snyder A, Shannon B, LaRossa G, Sachs R, Fotenos A. Molecular, structural, and functional characterization of Alzheimer's disease: Evidence for a relationship between default activity, amyloid, and memory. The Journal of Neuroscience. 2005;**25**:7709-7719

[6] Frolich L, Muller WE, Riederer P. Editorial: Siegfried Hoyer's concept of Alzheimer pathophysiology. Journal of Neural Transmission (Vienna). 2015;**122**(4):495-497

[7] Goyal MS, Vlassenko AG, Blazey TM, Su Y, Couture LE, Durbin TJ, et al. Loss of brain aerobic glycolysis in normal human aging. Cell Metabolism. 2017;**26**(2):353-60.e3

[8] Clark CM, Schneider JA, Bedell BJ, Beach TG, Bilker WB, Mintun MA, et al. Use of florbetapir-PET for imaging beta-amyloid pathology. JAMA. 2011;**305**(3):275-283

[9] Mathis CA, Wang Y, Klunk WE. Imaging beta-amyloid plaques and neurofibrillary tangles in the aging human brain. Current Pharmaceutical Design. 2004;**10**(13):1469-1492

[10] Chien DT, Bahri S, Szardenings AK, Walsh JC, Mu F, Su MY, et al. Early clinical PET imaging results with the novel PHF-tau radioligand [F-18]-T807. Journal of Alzheimer's Disease. 2013;**34**(2):457-468

[11] Jack CR Jr, Wiste HJ, Lesnick TG, Weigand SD, Knopman DS, Vemuri P, et al. Brain beta-amyloid load approaches a plateau. Neurology. 2013;**80**(10):890-896

[12] Jack CR Jr, Wiste HJ, Weigand SD, Therneau TM, Knopman DS, Lowe V, et al. Age-specific and sex-specific prevalence of cerebral beta-amyloidosis, tauopathy, and neurodegeneration in cognitively unimpaired individuals aged 50-95 years: A cross-sectional study. Lancet Neurology. 2017

[13] Sperling RA, Aisen PS, Beckett LA, Bennett DA, Craft S, Fagan AM, et al. Toward defining the preclinical stages of Alzheimer's disease: Recommendations from the National Institute on Aging-Alzheimer's Association workgroups on diagnostic guidelines for Alzheimer's disease. Alzheimers Dement. 2011;7(3):280-292

[14] Nelson PT, Alafuzoff I, Bigio EH, Bouras C, Braak H, Cairns NJ, et al. Correlation of Alzheimer disease neuropathologic changes with cognitive status: A review of the literature. Journal of Neuropathology and Experimental Neurology. 2012;**71**(5):362-381

[15] Bateman RJ, Xiong C, Benzinger TL, Fagan AM, Goate A, Fox NC, et al. Clinical and biomarker changes in dominantly inherited Alzheimer's

disease. The New England Journal of Medicine. 2012;**367**(9):795-804

[16] Wisniewski KE, Wisniewski HM, Wen GY. Occurrence of neuropathological changes and dementia of Alzheimer's disease in Down's syndrome. Annals of Neurology. 1985;**17**(3):278-282

[17] Braak H, Braak E. Neuropathological stageing of Alzheimer-related changes. Acta Neuropathologica. 1991;**82**(4):239-259

[18] Thal DR, Rub U, Orantes M, Braak H. Phases of A beta-deposition in the human brain and its relevance for the development of AD. Neurology. 2002;**58**(12):1791-1800

[19] Doraiswamy PM, Sperling RA, Coleman RE, Johnson KA, Reiman EM, Davis MD, et al. Amyloid-beta assessed by florbetapir F 18 PET and 18-month cognitive decline: A multicenter study. Neurology. 2012;**79**(16):1636-1644

[20] Minoshima S, Foster NL, Kuhl DE. Posterior cingulate cortex in Alzheimer's disease. Lancet. 1994;**344**(8926):895

[21] Minoshima S, Giordani B, Berent S, Frey KA, Foster NL, Kuhl DE. Metabolic reduction in the posterior cingulate cortex in very early Alzheimer's disease. Annals of Neurology. 1997;**42**(1):85-94

[22] Forster S, Grimmer T, Miederer I, Henriksen G, Yousefi BH, Graner P, et al. Regional expansion of hypometabolism in Alzheimer's disease follows amyloid deposition with temporal delay. Biological Psychiatry. 2012;**71**(9):792-797

[23] Rodrigue KM, Kennedy KM, Devous MD Sr, Rieck JR, Hebrank AC, Diaz-Arrastia R, et al. Beta-amyloid burden in healthy aging: Regional distribution and cognitive consequences. Neurology. 2012;**78**(6):387-395

[24] Palmqvist S, Scholl M, Strandberg O, Mattsson N, Stomrud E, Zetterberg H, et al. Earliest accumulation of beta-amyloid occurs within the default-mode network and concurrently affects brain connectivity. Nature Communications. 2017;**8**(1):1214

[25] Wirth M, Madison CM, Rabinovici GD, Oh H, Landau SM, Jagust WJ. Alzheimer's disease neurodegenerative biomarkers are associated with decreased cognitive function but not beta-amyloid in cognitively normal older individuals. The Journal of Neuroscience. 2013;**33**(13):5553-5563

[26] Wu L, Rowley J, Mohades S, Leuzy A, Dauar MT, Shin M, et al. Dissociation between brain amyloid deposition and metabolism in early mild cognitive impairment. PLoS One. 2012;**7**(10):e47905

[27] Dickerson BC, Bakkour A, Salat DH, Feczko E, Pacheco J, Greve DN, et al. The cortical signature of Alzheimer's disease: Regionally specific cortical thinning relates to symptom severity in very mild to mild AD dementia and is detectable in asymptomatic amyloid-positive individuals. Cerebral Cortex. 2009;**19**(3):497-510

[28] Becker JA, Hedden T, Carmasin J, Maye J, Rentz DM, Putcha D, et al. Amyloid-beta associated cortical thinning in clinically normal elderly. Annals of Neurology. 2011;**69**(6):1032-1042

[29] Arriagada PV, Growdon JH, Hedley-Whyte ET, Hyman BT. Neurofibrillary tangles but not senile plaques parallel duration and severity of Alzheimer's disease. Neurology. 1992;**42**(3 Pt 1): 631-639

[30] Braak H, Thal DR, Ghebremedhin E, Del Tredici K. Stages of the pathologic process in Alzheimer disease: Age categories from 1 to 100

years. Journal of Neuropathology and Experimental Neurology. 2011;**70**(11):960-969

[31] Hyman BT, Phelps CH, Beach TG, Bigio EH, Cairns NJ, Carrillo MC, et al. National Institute on Aging-Alzheimer's Association guidelines for the neuropathologic assessment of Alzheimer's disease. Alzheimers & Dementia. 2012;**8**(1):1-13

[32] Monsell SE, Kukull WA, Roher AE, Maarouf CL, Serrano G, Beach TG, et al. Characterizing apolipoprotein E epsilon4 carriers and noncarriers with the clinical diagnosis of mild to moderate Alzheimer dementia and minimal beta-amyloid peptide plaques. JAMA Neurology. 2015;**72**(10):1124-1131

[33] Crary JF, Trojanowski JQ, Schneider JA, Abisambra JF, Abner EL, Alafuzoff I, et al. Primary age-related tauopathy (PART): A common pathology associated with human aging. Acta Neuropathologica. 2014;**128**(6):755-766

[34] Scholl M, Lockhart SN, Schonhaut DR, O'Neil JP, Janabi M, Ossenkoppele R, et al. PET imaging of tau deposition in the aging human brain. Neuron. 2016;**89**(5):971-982

[35] Wang L, Benzinger TL, Su Y, Christensen J, Friedrichsen K, Aldea P, et al. Evaluation of tau imaging in staging Alzheimer disease and revealing interactions between beta-amyloid and tauopathy. JAMA Neurology. 2016;**73**(9):1070-1077

[36] Marks SM, Lockhart SN, Baker SL, Jagust WJ. Tau and beta-amyloid are associated with medial temporal lobe structure, function, and memory encoding in normal aging. The Journal of Neuroscience. 2017;**37**(12):3192-3201

[37] Ossenkoppele R, Schonhaut DR, Scholl M, Lockhart SN, Ayakta N, Baker SL, et al. Tau PET patterns mirror clinical and neuroanatomical variability in Alzheimer's disease. Brain. 2016;**139**(Pt 5):1551-1567

[38] Lehmann M, Ghosh PM, Madison C, Laforce R Jr, Corbetta-Rastelli C, Weiner MW, et al. Diverging patterns of amyloid deposition and hypometabolism in clinical variants of probable Alzheimer's disease. Brain. 2013;**136**(Pt 3):844-858

[39] Sepulcre J, Grothe MJ, d'Oleire Uquillas F, Ortiz-Terán L, Diez I, Yang H-S, et al. Neurogenetic contributions to amyloid beta and tau spreading in the human cortex. Nature Medicine. 2018;**24**(12):1910-1918

[40] Shulman GL, Fiez JA, Corbetta M, Buckner RL, Miezin FM, Raichle ME, et al. Common blood flow changes across visual tasks: I. Decreases in cerebral cortex. Journal of Cognitive Neuroscience. 1997;**9**(5):648-663

[41] Raichle ME, MacLeod AM, Snyder AZ, Powers WJ, Gusnard DA, Shulman GL. A default mode of brain function. Proceedings of the National Academy of Sciences of the United States of America. 2001;**98**(2):676-682

[42] Vincent JL, Patel GH, Fox MD, Snyder AZ, Baker JT, Van Essen DC, et al. Intrinsic functional architecture in the anaesthetized monkey brain. Nature. 2007;**447**(7140):83-86

[43] Christoff K, Irving ZC, Fox KCR, Spreng RN, Andrews-Hanna JR. Mind-wandering as spontaneous thought: A dynamic framework. Nature Reviews Neuroscience. 2016;**17**:718

[44] D'Argembeau A. On the role of the ventromedial prefrontal cortex in self-processing: The valuation hypothesis. Frontiers in Human Neuroscience. 2013;**7**:372

[45] Mason MF, Norton MI, Van Horn JD, Wegner DM, Grafton ST,

Macrae CN. Wandering minds: The default network and stimulus-independent thought. Science. 2007;**315**(5810):393-395

[46] Zald DH, Mattson DL, Pardo JV. Brain activity in ventromedial prefrontal cortex correlates with individual differences in negative affect. Proceedings of the National Academy of Sciences of the United States of America. 2002;**99**(4):2450-2454

[47] Hurliman E, Nagode JC, Pardo JV. Double dissociation of exteroceptive and interoceptive feedback systems in the orbital and ventromedial prefrontal cortex of humans. The Journal of Neuroscience. 2005;**25**(18):4641-4648

[48] Biswal B, Yetkin FZ, Haughton VM, Hyde JS. Functional connectivity in the motor cortex of resting human brain using echo-planar MRI. Magnetic Resonance in Medicine. 1995;**34**(4):537-541

[49] Greicius MD, Krasnow B, Reiss AL, Menon V. Functional connectivity in the resting brain: A network analysis of the default mode hypothesis. Proceedings of the National Academy of Sciences of the United States of America. 2003;**100**(1):253-258

[50] Hahn A, Wadsak W, Windischberger C, Baldinger P, Hoflich AS, Losak J, et al. Differential modulation of the default mode network via serotonin-1a receptors. Proceedings of the National Academy of Sciences of the United States of America. 2012;**109**(7):2619-2624

[51] Harrison BJ, Pujol J, Lopez-Sola M, Hernandez-Ribas R, Deus J, Ortiz H, et al. Consistency and functional specialization in the default mode brain network. Proceedings of the National Academy of Sciences of the United States of America. 2008;**105**(28):9781-9786

[52] Jones DT, Vemuri P, Murphy MC, Gunter JL, Senjem ML, Machulda MM, et al. Non-stationarity in the "resting brain's" modular architecture. PLoS One. 2012;**7**(6):e39731

[53] Damoiseaux JS, Rombouts SARB, Barkhof F, Scheltens P, Stam CJ, Smith SM, et al. Consistent resting-state networks across healthy subjects. Proceedings of the National Academy of Sciences of the United States of America. 2006;**103**:13848-13853

[54] Esposito R, Cilli F, Pieramico V, Ferretti A, Macchia A, Tommasi M, et al. Acute effects of modafinil on brain resting state networks in young healthy subjects. PLoS One. 2013;**8**(7):e69224

[55] Cha J, Jo HJ, Gibson WS, Lee J-M. Functional organization of the human posterior cingulate cortex, revealed by multiple connectivity-based parcellation methods. Human Brain Mapping. 2017;**38**(6):2808-2818

[56] Glasser MF, Coalson TS, Robinson EC, Hacker CD, Harwell J, Yacoub E, et al. A multi-modal parcellation of human cerebral cortex. Nature. 2016;**536**(7615):171-178

[57] Braga RM, Buckner RL. Parallel interdigitated distributed networks within the individual estimated by intrinsic functional connectivity. Neuron. 2017;**95**(2):457-71.e5

[58] Mormino EC, Smiljic A, Hayenga AO, Onami SH, Greicius MD, Rabinovici GD, et al. Relationships between beta-amyloid and functional connectivity in different components of the default mode network in aging. Cerebral Cortex.**21**(10):2399-2407

[59] Brier MR, Thomas JB, Snyder AZ, Wang L, Fagan AM, Benzinger T, et al. Unrecognized preclinical Alzheimer disease confounds rs-fcMRI studies of normal aging. Neurology. 2014;**83**(18):1613-1619

[60] Greicius MD, Srivastava G, Reiss AL, Menon V. Default-mode network activity distinguishes Alzheimer's disease from healthy aging: Evidence from functional MRI. Proceedings of the National Academy of Sciences of the United States of America. 2004;**101**(13):4637-4642

[61] Vincent JL, Snyder AZ, Fox MD, Shannon BJ, Andrews JR, Raichle ME, et al. Coherent spontaneous activity identifies a hippocampal-parietal memory network. Journal of Neurophysiology. 2006;**96**(6):3517-3531

[62] Qin S, Duan X, Supekar K, Chen H, Chen T, Menon V. Large-scale intrinsic functional network organization along the long axis of the human medial temporal lobe. Brain Structure & Function. 2016;**221**(6):3237-3258

[63] Ward AM, Schultz AP, Huijbers W, Van Dijk KR, Hedden T, Sperling RA. The parahippocampal gyrus links the default-mode cortical network with the medial temporal lobe memory system. Human Brain Mapping. 2014;**35**(3):1061-1073

[64] Andrews-Hanna JR, Reidler JS, Huang C, Buckner RL. Evidence for the default network's role in spontaneous cognition. Journal of Neurophysiology.**104**(1):322-335

[65] Huijbers W, Pennartz CM, Cabeza R, Daselaar SM. The hippocampus is coupled with the default network during memory retrieval but not during memory encoding. PLoS One. 2011;**6**(4):e17463

[66] Sperling RA, Laviolette PS, O'Keefe K, O'Brien J, Rentz DM, Pihlajamaki M, et al. Amyloid deposition is associated with impaired default network function in older persons without dementia. Neuron. 2009;**63**(2):178-188

[67] Castro MA, Beltran FA, Brauchi S, Concha II. A metabolic switch in brain: Glucose and lactate metabolism modulation by ascorbic acid. Journal of Neurochemistry. 2009;**110**(2):423-440

[68] Erbsloh F, Bernsmeier A, Hillesheim H. The glucose consumption of the brain & its dependence on the liver. Archiv für Psychiatrie und Nervenkrankheiten, vereinigt mit Zeitschrift für die gesamte Neurologie und Psychiatrie. 1958;**196**(6):611-626

[69] Vlassenko AG, Gordon BA, Goyal MS, Su Y, Blazey TM, Durbin TJ, et al. Aerobic glycolysis and tau deposition in preclinical Alzheimer's disease. Neurobiology of Aging. 2018;**67**:95-98

[70] Kety S. A biologist examines the mind and behavior. Science. 1960;**132**(3443):1861-1867

[71] Fox PT, Raichle ME, Mintun MA, Dence C. Nonoxidative glucose consumption during focal physiologic neural activity. Science. 1988;**241**(4864):462-464

[72] Mangold R, Sokoloff L, Conner E, Kleinerman J, Therman PO, Kety SS. The effects of sleep and lack of sleep on the cerebral circulation and metabolism of normal young men. The Journal of Clinical Investigation. 1955;**34**(7, Part 1):1092-1100

[73] Vaishnavi SN, Vlassenko AG, Rundle MM, Snyder AZ, Mintun MA, Raichle ME. Regional aerobic glycolysis in the human brain. Proceedings of the National Academy of Sciences of the United States of America. 2010;**107**(41):17757-17762

[74] Vlassenko AG, Vaishnavi SN, Couture L, Sacco D, Shannon BJ, Mach RH, et al. Spatial correlation between brain aerobic glycolysis and amyloid-beta (abeta) deposition. Proceedings of the National Academy of Sciences of the United States of America. 2010;**107**(41):17763-17767

[75] Bauernfeind AL, Barks SK, Duka T, Grossman LI, Hof PR, Sherwood CC. Aerobic glycolysis in the primate brain: Reconsidering the implications for growth and maintenance. Brain Structure & Function. 2014;**219**(4):1149-1167

[76] Goyal MS, Hawrylycz M, Miller JA, Snyder AZ, Raichle ME. Aerobic glycolysis in the human brain is associated with development and neotenous gene expression. Cell Metabolism. 2014;**19**(1):49-57

[77] Shannon BJ, Vaishnavi SN, Vlassenko AG, Shimony JS, Rutlin J, Raichle ME. Brain aerobic glycolysis and motor adaptation learning. Proceedings of the National Academy of Sciences of the United States of America. 2016;**113**(26):E3782-E3791

[78] Musiek ES, Holtzman DM. Three dimensions of the amyloid hypothesis: Time, space and 'wingmen'. Nature Neuroscience. 2015;**18**(6):800-806

[79] Potter R, Patterson BW, Elbert DL, Ovod V, Kasten T, Sigurdson W, et al. Increased in vivo amyloid-beta42 production, exchange, and loss in presenilin mutation carriers. Science Translational Medicine. 2013;**5**(189):189ra77

[80] Jonsson T, Atwal JK, Steinberg S, Snaedal J, Jonsson PV, Bjornsson S, et al. A mutation in APP protects against Alzheimer's disease and age-related cognitive decline. Nature. 2012;**488**(7409):96-99

[81] Bero AW, Yan P, Roh JH, Cirrito JR, Stewart FR, Raichle ME, et al. Neuronal activity regulates the regional vulnerability to amyloid-beta deposition. Nature Neuroscience. 2011;**14**(6):750-756

[82] Cirrito JR, Yamada KA, Finn MB, Sloviter RS, Bales KR, May PC, et al. Synaptic activity regulates interstitial fluid amyloid-beta levels in vivo. Neuron. 2005;**48**(6):913-922

[83] Leal SL, Landau SM, Bell RK, Jagust WJ. Hippocampal activation is associated with longitudinal amyloid accumulation and cognitive decline. eLife. 2017;**6**:e22978

[84] Kanekiyo T, Xu H, Bu G. APOE and A-beta in Alzheimer's disease: Accidental encounters or partners? Neuron. 2014;**81**(4):740-754

[85] Mawuenyega KG, Sigurdson W, Ovod V, Munsell L, Kasten T, Morris JC, et al. Decreased clearance of CNS beta-amyloid in Alzheimer's disease. Science. 2010;**330**(6012):1774

[86] Ibanez V, Pietrini P, Alexander GE, Furey ML, Teichberg D, Rajapakse JC, et al. Regional glucose metabolic abnormalities are not the result of atrophy in Alzheimer's disease. Neurology. 1998;**50**(6):1585-1593

[87] Davatzikos C, Xu F, An Y, Fan Y, Resnick SM. Longitudinal progression of Alzheimer's-like patterns of atrophy in normal older adults: The SPARE-AD index. Brain. 2009;**132**(Pt 8):2026-2035

[88] Beason-Held L, Kraut M, Resnick S. I: Longitudinal changes in aging brain function. Neurobiology of Aging. 2008;**29**:483-496

[89] McDonald CR, McEvoy LK, Gharapetian L, Fennema-Notestine C, Hagler DJ Jr, Holland D, et al. Regional rates of neocortical atrophy from normal aging to early Alzheimer disease. Neurology. 2009;**73**(6):457-465

[90] Rowe CC, Ng S, Ackermann U, Gong SJ, Pike K, Savage G, et al. Imaging beta-amyloid burden in aging and dementia. Neurology. 2007;**68**(20):1718-1725

[91] Reiman EM, Chen K, Liu X, Bandy D, Yu M, Lee W, et al. Fibrillar

amyloid-beta burden in cognitively normal people at 3 levels of genetic risk for Alzheimer's disease. Proceedings of the National Academy of Sciences of the United States of America. 2009;**106**(16):6820-6825

[92] Fleisher AS, Chen K, Liu X, Ayutyanont N, Roontiva A, Thiyyagura P, et al. Apolipoprotein E epsilon4 and age effects on florbetapir positron emission tomography in healthy aging and Alzheimer disease. Neurobiology of Aging. 2013;34(1):1-12

[93] Reiman EM, Chen K, Alexander GE, Caselli RJ, Bandy D, Osborne D, et al. Functional brain abnormalities in young adults at genetic risk for late-onset Alzheimer's dementia. Proceedings of the National Academy of Sciences of the United States of America. 2004;**101**(1):284-289

[94] Liu L, Caselli RJ. Age stratification corrects bias in estimated hazard of APOE genotype for Alzheimer's disease. Alzheimer's & Dementia: Translational Research and Clinical Interventions. (New York, N. Y.). 2018;**4**:602-608

[95] Sheline YI, Morris JC, Snyder AZ, Price JL, Yan Z, D'Angelo G, et al. APOE4 allele disrupts resting state fMRI connectivity in the absence of amyloid plaques or decreased CSF abeta42. The Journal of Neuroscience. 2010;**30**(50):17035-17040

[96] Martin AJ, Friston KJ, Colebatch JG, Frackowiak RS. Decreases in regional cerebral blood flow with normal aging. Journal of Cerebral Blood Flow and Metabolism. 1991;**11**(4):684-689

[97] Moeller JR, Ishikawa T, Dhawan V, Spetsieris P, Mandel F, Alexander GE, et al. The metabolic topography of normal aging. Journal of Cerebral Blood Flow and Metabolism. 1996;**16**(3):385-398

[98] Schultz SK, O'Leary DS, Boles Ponto LL, Watkins GL, Hichwa RD, Andreasen NC. Age-related changes in regional cerebral blood flow among young to mid-life adults. Neuroreport. 1999;**10**(12):2493-2496

[99] Pardo JV, Lee JT, Sheikh S, Surerus-Johnson C, Shah H, Munch K. Where the brain grows old: Decline in anterior cingulate and medial prefrontal function with normal aging. NeuroImage. 2007;**35**:1231-1237

[100] Vaidya JG, Paradiso S, Boles Ponto LL, McCormick LM, Robinson RG. Aging, grey matter, and blood flow in the anterior cingulate cortex. NeuroImage. 2007;**37**(4):1346-1353

[101] Shen X, Liu H, Hu Z, Hu H, Shi P. The relationship between cerebral glucose metabolism and age: Report of a large brain PET data set. PLoS One. 2012;**7**(12):e51517

[102] Andrews-Hanna JR, Snyder AZ, Vincent JL, Lustig C, Head D, Raichle ME, et al. Disruption of large-scale brain systems in advanced aging. Neuron. 2007;**56**(5):924-935

[103] Jones DT, Machulda MM, Vemuri P, McDade EM, Zeng G, Senjem ML, et al. Age-related changes in the default mode network are more advanced in Alzheimer disease. Neurology. 2011;**77**(16):1524-1531

[104] Sowell ER, Peterson BS, Thompson PM, Welcome SE, Henkenius AL, Toga AW. Mapping cortical change across the human life span. Nature Neuroscience. 2003;**6**(3):309-315

[105] Salat DH, Buckner RL, Snyder AZ, Greve DN, Desikan RS, Busa E, et al. Thinning of the cerebral cortex in aging. Cerebral Cortex. 2004;**14**(7):721-730

[106] Mann SL, Hazlett EA, Byne W, Hof PR, Buchsbaum MS, Cohen BH,

et al. Anterior and posterior cingulate cortex volume in healthy adults: Effects of aging and gender differences. Brain Research. 2011;**1401**:18-29

[107] Schultz SA, Gordon BA, Mishra S, Su Y, Perrin RJ, Cairns NJ, et al. Widespread distribution of tauopathy in preclinical Alzheimer's disease. Neurobiology of Aging. 2018;**72**:177-185

[108] Gefen T, Peterson M, Papastefan ST, Martersteck A, Whitney K, Rademaker A, et al. Morphometric and histologic substrates of cingulate integrity in elders with exceptional memory capacity. The Journal of Neuroscience. 2015;**35**(4):1781-1791

[109] Fjell AM, Westlye LT, Grydeland H, Amlien I, Espeseth T, Reinvang I, et al. Accelerating cortical thinning: Unique to dementia or universal in aging? Cerebral Cortex. 2014;**24**(4):919-934

[110] Liu Y, Julkunen V, Paajanen T, Westman E, Wahlund L-O, Aitken A, et al. Education increases reserve against Alzheimer's disease—Evidence from structural MRI analysis. Neuroradiology. 2012:929-938

[111] Arenaza-Urquijo EM, Landeau B, La Joie R, Mevel K, Mezenge F, Perrotin A, et al. Relationships between years of education and gray matter volume, metabolism and functional connectivity in healthy elders. NeuroImage. 2013;**83**:450-457

[112] Colcombe SJ, Erickson KI, Scalf PE, Kim JS, Prakash R, McAuley E, et al. Aerobic exercise training increases brain volume in aging humans. The Journals of Gerontology. Series A, Biological Sciences and Medical Sciences. 2006;**61**(11):1166-1170

[113] Klunk WE, Price JC, Mathis CA, Tsopelas ND, Lopresti BJ, Ziolko SK, et al. Amyloid deposition begins in the striatum of presenilin-1 mutation carriers from two unrelated pedigrees. The Journal of Neuroscience. 2007;**27**(23):6174-6184

[114] Remes AM, Laru L, Tuominen H, Aalto S, Kemppainen N, Mononen H, et al. Carbon 11-labeled Pittsburgh compound B positron emission tomographic amyloid imaging in patients with APP locus duplication. Archives of Neurology. 2008;**65**(4):540-544

[115] Villemagne VL, Ataka S, Mizuno T, Brooks WS, Wada Y, Kondo M, et al. High striatal amyloid beta-peptide deposition across different autosomal Alzheimer disease mutation types. Archives of Neurology. 2009;**66**(12):1537-1544

[116] Sun L, Zhou R, Yang G, Shi Y. Analysis of 138 pathogenic mutations in presenilin-1 on the in vitro production of abeta42 and abeta40 peptides by gamma-secretase. Proceedings of the National Academy of Sciences of the United States of America. 2017;**114**(4):E476-EE85

[117] Lao PJ, Betthauser TJ, Hillmer AT, Price JC, Klunk WE, Mihaila I, et al. The effects of normal aging on amyloid-beta deposition in nondemented adults with down syndrome as imaged by carbon 11-labeled Pittsburgh compound B. Alzheimers Dement. 2016;**12**(4):380-390

[118] Ballatore C, Lee VM, Trojanowski JQ. Tau-mediated neurodegeneration in Alzheimer's disease and related disorders. Nature Reviews Neuroscience. 2007;**8**(9):663-672

[119] Braak H, Del Tredici K. The pathological process underlying Alzheimer's disease in individuals under thirty. Acta Neuropathologica. 2011;**121**(2):171-181

[120] Shi Y, Yamada K, Liddelow SA, Smith ST, Zhao L, Luo W, et al. APOE4 markedly exacerbates tau-mediated neurodegeneration in a mouse model of tauopathy. Nature. 2017;**549**(7673):523-527

[121] Khan UA, Liu L, Provenzano FA, Berman DE, Profaci CP, Sloan R, Mayeux R, Duff KE, Small SA. Molecular drivers and cortical spread of lateral entorhinal cortex dysfunction in preclinical Alzheimer's disease. Nature Neuroscience. 2014;17(2):303-311

[122] Mintun MA, Vlassenko AG, Rundle MM, Raichle ME. Increased lactate/pyruvate ratio augments blood flow in physiologically activated human brain. Proceedings of the National Academy of Sciences of the United States of America. 2004;**101**(2):659-664

[123] Fernandez-Moncada I, Ruminot I, Robles-Maldonado D, Alegria K, Deitmer JW, Barros LF. Neuronal control of astrocytic respiration through a variant of the Crabtree effect. Proceedings of the National Academy of Sciences of the United States of America. 2018;**115**(7):1623-1628

[124] Suzuki A, Stern SA, Bozdagi O, Huntley GW, Walker RH, Magistretti PJ, et al. Astrocyte-neuron lactate transport is required for long-term memory formation. Cell. 2011;**144**(5):810-823

[125] Madsen PL, Hasselbalch SG, Hagemann LP, Olsen KS, Bülow J, Holm S, et al. Persistent resetting of the cerebral oxygen/glucose uptake ratio by brain activation: Evidence obtained with the Kety—Schmidt technique. Journal of Cerebral Blood Flow and Metabolism. 1995;**15**(3):485-491

[126] Nakamura A, Cuesta P, Fernández A, Arahata Y, Iwata K, Kuratsubo I, et al. Electromagnetic signatures of the preclinical and prodromal stages of Alzheimer's disease. Brain. 2018;**141**(5):1470-1485

[127] Jones DT, Knopman DS, Gunter JL, Graff-Radford J, Vemuri P, Boeve BF, et al. Cascading network failure across the Alzheimer's disease spectrum. Brain. 2016;**139**(Pt 2):547-562

Chapter 3

Mitochondria and Alzheimer's Disease: An Electron Microscopy Study

Stavros J. Baloyannis

Abstract

Alzheimer's disease is a progressive, irreversible presenile or senile neurodegenerative disorder, implicating mainly the mental faculties, characterized by decline of memory and judgment, learning impairment, loss of professional skills and verbal capacities, alterations of social behavior, decline of motor skills and eventual disarrangement of the autonomic equilibrium. Among the pathogenetic factors, oxidative stress and mitochondrial dysfunction may play an essential role. Alterations of mitochondria may enhance amyloid toxicity, which in turn may aggravate mitochondrial dysfunction. We describe ultrastructural alterations of mitochondria in the soma of neurons, in axons, dendritic profiles and synaptic terminals, in astrocytes in early cases of Alzheimer's disease on various areas of the cerebral and the cerebellar cortex, the hippocampus, the hypothalamus, the mammillary bodies and the medial geniculate body. The morphological and morphometric study of the mitochondria revealed an impressive polymorphism at any area of the brain. The mitochondria demonstrated variation of size and shape, fragmentation of the cristae and marked changes of their structure. The most dramatic mitochondrial alterations were observed in dendritic profiles, spines and synaptic terminals. A substantial number of astrocytes demonstrated mitochondrial alterations, which coexisted with fragmentation of Golgi apparatus and dilatation of the cisternae of the smooth endoplasmic reticulum. On the basis of our observations, we feel that therapeutic strategies aiming at protecting the mitochondria might be beneficial in the treatment of early cases of AD.

Keywords: Alzheimer's disease, mitochondria, Golgi apparatus, astrocytes, synapses, electron microscopy

1. Introduction

Alzheimer's disease (AD) is one of the most enigmatic and multidimensional neurodegenerative diseases of the brain. The high incidence in aging, the ongoing number of the patients and the social, humanitarian and economic impact of the disease [1], as well as the irreversible course of the disease, the failure of therapeutic interventions [2] and the fatal outcome impose on the neuroscientists and the society a combined attempt for the amelioration of the quality of life of the patients at least by the reduction of risk factors in the initial stages of the disease [3].

The clinical manifestation of Alzheimer's disease, starting from the inability to encode new memories, includes progressive and irreversible cognitive decline, affecting memory and judgment, loss of professional skills and verbal capacities, impairment of learning new informations and gradual disarrangement of the social behavior [4, 5] resulting in isolation of the patient in the framework of an obvious functional incapacity, encountering in vegetative state eventually.

The neuropathological background of AD mostly consists of selective neuronal loss [6, 7], substantial morphological and morphometric alterations of the synapses [8–11], marked mitochondrial alterations, even in the initial stages of the disease [12, 13], tau pathology [14] resulting in the formation of neurofibrillary tangles (NFT) by the accumulation of hyperphosphorylated tau protein [15], many inflammatory phenomena, alterations of brain capillaries [16] and various extensive extracellular deposits of Aβ peptide's polymers, in the form of polymorphic neuritic plaques, [17, 18].

Pathological alterations of the organelles in the soma, the axons, the dendrites and the synapses of neurons are observed in electron microscopy, even in the initial stage of the disease [19] in areas with minimal typical Alzheimer's pathology, namely aggregations of Aβ peptide and neurofibrillary tangles. The majority of the alterations of the organelles in Alzheimer's disease particularly concern the Golgi complex [19], the microtubules, the synaptic vesicles and mostly the mitochondria [20–22].

The etiopathology of the sporadic cases of Alzheimer's disease remains a real problem in spite of the multidimensional extensive ongoing research in the last decades [23, 24] on the crucial fields of genetics [25, 26], molecular biology [27, 28], neuropathology [29, 30], neuroimmunology [31, 32], pathophysiology [33], neuroimaging [34] and neurochemistry [35–38].

The pathogenetic mechanisms embrace a diverse range of hypotheses which attempt to decipher the real cause of memory and reasoning decline in AD. Among the many hypothesis, the most mattering are (a) the amyloid hypothesis [39, 40], (b) the metabolic and synaptic dysfunction hypothesis [41], (c) the hypothesis of translational neurodegeneration [42], (d) the tau hypothesis [43], (e) the hypothesis of neuroinflammation [44], (f) the cholinergic hypothesis [45], (g) the oxidative stress [46], (h) the vascular hypothesis [47, 48], (i) the glucose hypometabolism hypothesis [49], (j) the autoimmune hypothesis [50], (k) the endocrine hypothesis [51, 52], (l) the mitochondrial dysfunction [53, 54] and (m) the Golgi complex hypothesis [55–57].

Many of those hypotheses are basely interrelated, such as the amyloid hypothesis and the oxidative stress ones [58, 59], the amyloid and the tau hypothesis [60], the oxidative stress and the mitochondrial dysfunction [61], the mitochondrial dysfunction, energy deficiency and oxidative stress [61, 62], the mitochondria dysfunction and the synaptic pathology [22, 63], the tau pathology and the vascular hypothesis [64], the cholinergic dysfunction and the amyloid hypothesis [65], amyloid, tau and neurodegeneration hypothesis [66], the mitochondria and the dendritic hypothesis [67–69] and the immune reactions, microglia, tau, Aβ peptide, lipid processing and neurodegeneration hypothesis [70–73].

Mitochondria hypothesis advocates in favor of the important role that mitochondrial dysfunction may play in the early stages of Alzheimer's disease [21] by inducing energy deficiency and oxidative stress [22], which would be associated with β-amyloid (Aβ) neurotoxicity. It is well known that mitochondria, which has been defined as organelles in tissue culture since 1914 [74] are normally involved in aging process [75–77], since mitochondrial function declines as the age advances, resulting in decrease of ATP production and increase of free oxygen radicals formation, given that ATP synthase is located in the inner mitochondrial membrane, playing a key role in the energy homeostasis of the cell.

In addition, morphological alterations of mitochondria, resulting in deficiency of mitochondrial electron transport proteins, with considerable consequences upon the energy supply of nerve cells have been described in Alzheimer's disease and other degenerative conditions of the brain [12, 21, 78, 79], which are also associated with oxidative stress [80].

It is also particularly noticeable that morphological abnormalities of mitochondria are seen in neurons lacking neurofibrillary tangles [12] suggesting that mitochondrial degeneration might be among the earliest signs of Alzheimer's morphological alterations.

The fact that maternal influence seems to be a risk factor for Alzheimer's disease morbidity, according to epidemiologic studies [81, 82], and to combined neuropsychological and neuroimaging investigations [83] plead in favor of the substantial role that mitochondria may also play in the pathogenetic cascade of Alzheimer's disease.

In this perspective article, we attempted to describe the ultrastructural alterations of mitochondria in various neocortical and subcortical areas of the brain of patients who suffered from Alzheimer's disease at the early stages.

2. Material and methods

2.1 Material

This electron microscope study is based on examination of 25 brains obtained at autopsy 2–7 hours after death at a room temperature of 40°C. All of the brains were derived from patients aged 55–80 years, who have had a history of dementia, which was definitely diagnosed 1 or 3 years prior to the end of their life.

The patients fulfilled on repeated clinical examinations and assessments all the psychological, psychiatric and neurological criteria of AD [84–86]. The patients have had 18 years of education, and had a fluency in their native language, two of them being also bilingual with equal fluency in both of the languages. The usual diagnostic assessment was based on the medical history, the physical examination, including cardiological investigation, neurological examination, psychiatric evaluation and detailed neuropsychological testing.

The cognition of the patients was evaluated by battery of neuropsychological testing [87], including mini mental state examination (MMSE) [88, 89], dementia rating scale (DRS) [90, 91], ADAS-COX test [92, 93] and the brief memory executive test (BMET) [94].

All the patients underwent an EEG examination and a carotid examination by duplex Doppler. Neuroimaging was performed including computerized tomography (CT), magnetic resonance imaging (MRI) of the brain and a single-photon emission computed tomography (SPECT) [95]. All the methods of clinical and laboratory investigations were evocative for Alzheimer's disease. The patients passed away due to heart arrest.

In addition, we dissected and examined in electron microscopy 25 brains, which were unremarkable from the neuropathological point of view, derived from apparently healthy individuals of the same age range with the AD patients, using them as normal controls.

2.2 Methods

2.2.1 Electron microscopy

Multiple samples of a small size (2 × 2 × 2 mm) were excised from the hippocampus, the prefrontal area of the cortex, the superior parietal lobe, the occipital pole, the visual cortex, the Hessl gyri of the temporal neocortex, the vermis of the cerebellum and the cerebellar hemispheres, the hypothalamus, the mammillary bodies and the medial geniculate bodies. The samples were selected bilaterally and immersed directly in Sotelo's fixing solution [96], composed of 1% paraformaldehyde, 2.5% glutaraldehyde in cacodylate buffer 0.1 M, adjusted at pH 7.35.

Then all the specimens were post fixed in 1% osmium tetroxide for 30 min at a room temperature of 18°C and dehydrated in graded alcohol solutions and in propylene oxide twice. After dehydration, the specimens were embedded in araldite mixture and cut in ultrathin sections by a Reichert ultratome.

The sections were placed on the grids where they were contrasted with uranyl acetate and lead citrate, and studied in a Zeiss electron microscope of the type 9aS.

The study electron microscopy examination was particularly focused on the morphology of the organelles, mainly on the mitochondria of neurons and astrocytes. In addition, the Golgi complex, the endoplasmic reticulum, the endosomes, the dendritic profiles, the spines, the axons, the axonic collaterals and the synaptic components were studies in all of the sections.

The morphometric estimation was carried out on micrographs of a standard magnification of 56,000×. The analysis of each macrograph was performed with an image analyzer. The surface area of mitochondria as well as the volume and the circularity ratio (CR) were calculated on a total of 8000 mitochondria.

The statistical analysis of the data was evaluated by Student t tests.

3. Results

The ultrastructural study of the mitochondria revealed an impressive polymorphism at any area of the brain. The mitochondria demonstrated a wide variation of size and shape in the soma, the axons, the dendrites and the synaptic terminals in the majority of the neurons (**Figure 1**). The majority of the mitochondria demonstrated fragmentation of the cristae and obvious disarrangement of their interior

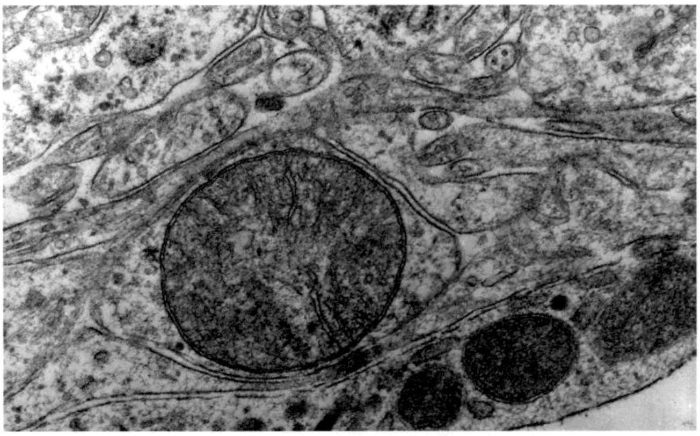

Figure 1.
Large round mitochondrion in a dendritic profile in the molecular layer of the cerebellum in a case of AD. Electron micrograph Mag. 248,000×.

structure (**Figures 1** and **2**). The mitochondria in the presynaptic terminals were either small and round with few cristae (**Figure 3**) or very large showing disruption of the cristae (**Figure 4**).

It should be underlined that in areas of the brain with minimal Alzheimer's pathology, such as the cerebellum, the visual, the acoustic cortex, the mammillary bodies and the hypothalamus, mitochondria demonstrated obvious morphological alterations. Very large mitochondria were observed in the soma and the dendritic profiles of Purkinje cells (**Figure 5**), in the granule cells (**Figure 6**) as well as in the climbing fibers, the mossy fibers and the synaptic terminals of parallel fibers (**Figure 7**). Large number of small mitochondria with disruption of cristae was observed in the visual cortex (**Figure 8**) and the acoustic cortex (**Figure 9**).

Mitochondrial alterations were also observed in many synaptic profiles in the suprachiasmatic and the paraventricular hypothalamic nuclei of AD brains (**Figure 10**).

The morphometric estimation of the mitochondria in the soma, the dendrites and the dendritic spines of a considerable number of neurons of the suprachiasmatic nucleus in AD brains revealed that they have an average diameter of 440 ± 250 nm and a mean axial ratio of 1.7 ± 0.2 [97].

The polymorphism of the mitochondria was the most frequent finding at any studied area of the cortex of the brain hemispheres, the cerebellum and the subcortical structures. Small round mitochondria intermixed with very large ones with disarrangement of the cristae and accumulation of fibrillary elements (**Figure 11**) or dense osmiophilic material (**Figure 12**). The mitochondria in the dendritic profiles and the synaptic terminals at the prefrontal cortex were large occupying the majority of the volume of the synaptic component (**Figure 1**). Large mitochondria were also observed in axonic collaterals among the myelinated fibers at the prefrontal and the parietal cortices (**Figure 13**). Small mitochondria were frequently observed in association with Golgi complex alterations in the soma of neurons and astrocytes (**Figure 14**).

A substantial number of astrocytes demonstrated small or very large mitochondria with disruption of the cristae in association with dilated cisternae of the smooth endoplasmic reticulum (**Figure 15**). Small mitochondria were also observed

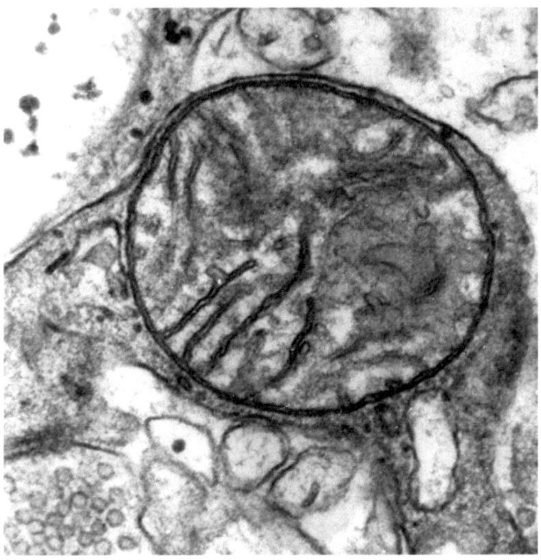

Figure 2.
Large mitochondrion in a postsynaptic terminal in the molecular layer of the cerebellum in a case of AD. The disruption of the mitochondrial cristae is obvious. Electron micrograph Mag. 248,000×.

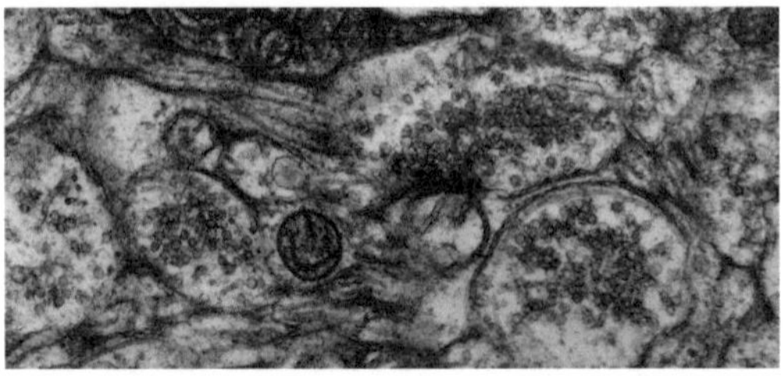

Figure 3.
Small round mitochondria in Purkinje cell dendritic spines (postsynaptic components) in the molecular layer of the cerebellum in a case of AD. Electron micrograph Mag. 248,000×.

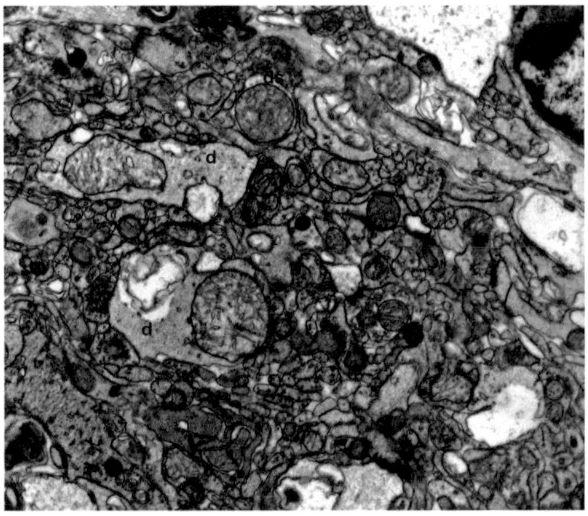

Figure 4.
Very large mitochondria in dendritic profiles (d) and dendritic spines (ds) in the molecular layer of the cerebellum in a case of AD. The disruption of the mitochondrial cristae and the disarrangement of the interior structure are obvious. Electron micrograph Mag. 56,000×.

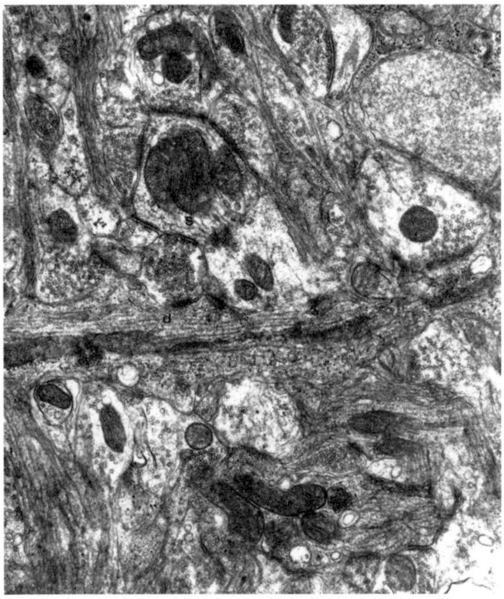

Figure 5.
Very elongated and large mitochondria in dendritic profiles (d) and dendritic spines (ds) in the molecular layer of the vermis of the cerebellum in a case of AD. The presynaptic terminals of the parallel fibers (pf) contain small round dense mitochondria. Electron micrograph Mag. 124,000×.

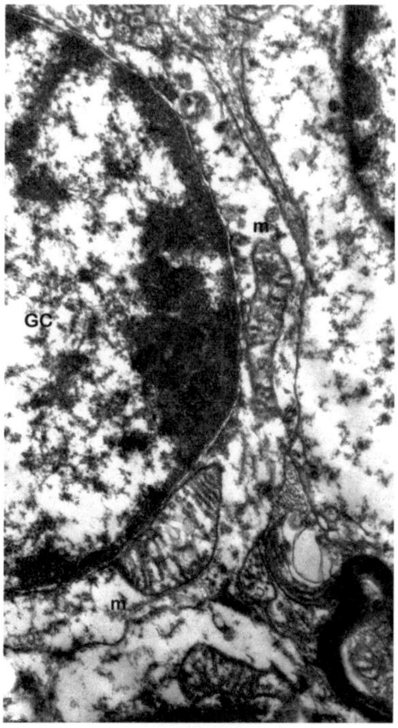

Figure 6.
Large abnormal mitochondria (m) in the perikaryon of a granule cell (GC) of the vermis of the cerebellum in a case of AD. Electron micrograph Mag. 124,000×.

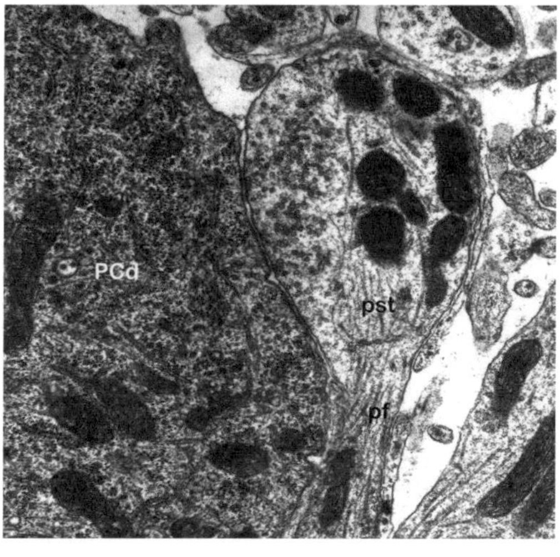

Figure 7.
Small dense mitochondria in a presynaptic terminal (pst) of a parallel fiber (pf) in contact with a large dendritic branch of Purkinje cell (PCd) in the molecular layer of the left cerebellar hemisphere in a case of AD. Electron micrograph Mag. 124,000×.

in oligodendrocytes in the subcortical white mater in association with dilated cisternae of the smooth endoplasmic reticulum and alterations of the Golgi complex (**Figure 16**).

The dendritic spines of the cortical neurons were dramatically reduced in number and size and most of the presynaptic terminals included small round and dense mitochondria and were also characterized by the dramatic poverty of the synaptic vesicles (**Figure 17**), a finding advocating in favor of a previous concept that the

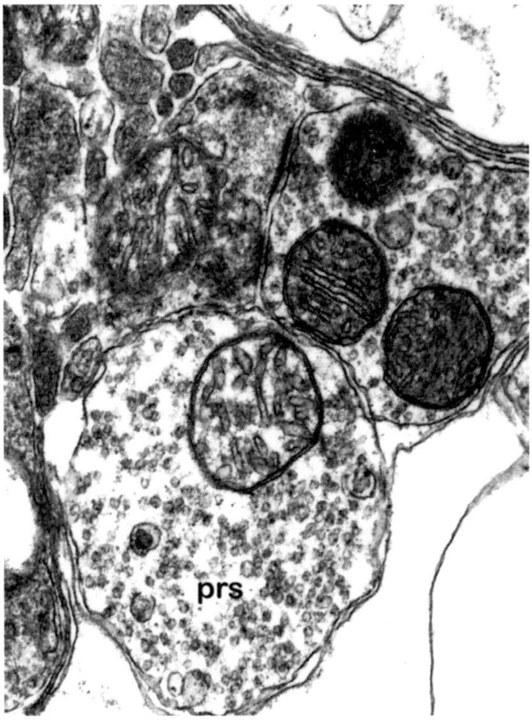

Figure 8.
Mitochondria with obvious disruption of the cristae in presynaptic terminal (prs) in the visual cortex in a case of AD. Electron micrograph Mag. 124,000×.

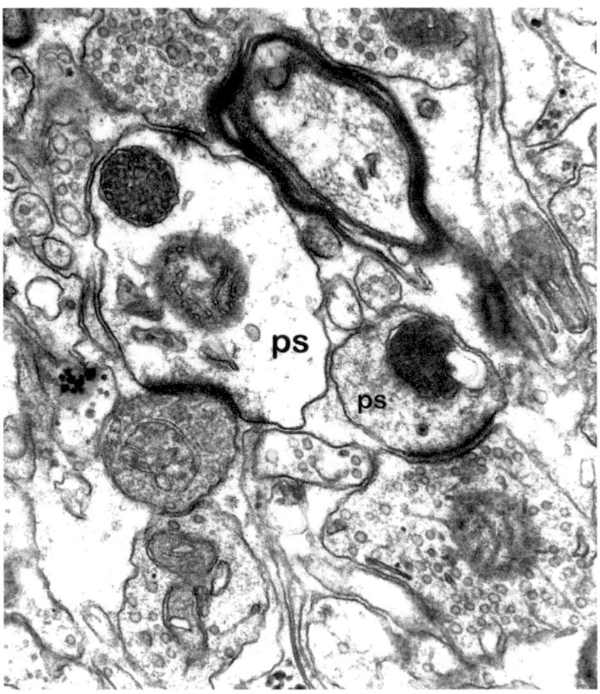

Figure 9.
Small dense mitochondria in postsynaptic terminal (ps) in the acoustic cortex in a case of AD. Electron micrograph Mag. 124,000×.

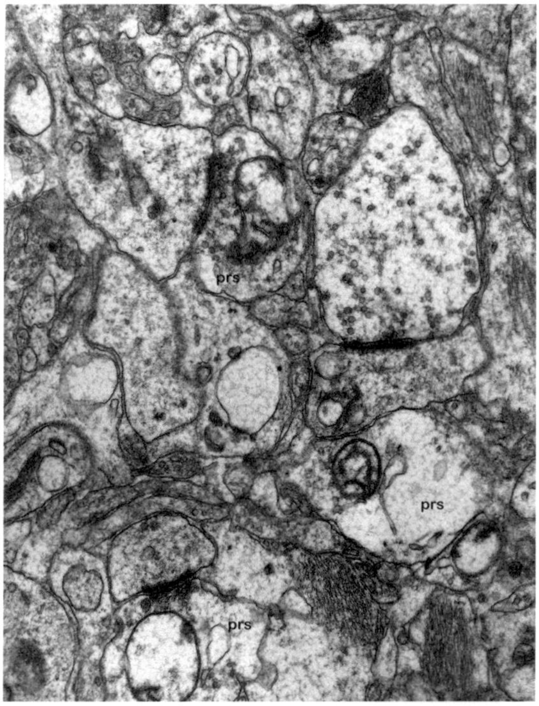

Figure 10.
Small abnormal mitochondria with disruption of the cristae and disintegration of the interior structure in the suprachiasmatic nucleus of the hypothalamus in a case of AD. Electron micrograph Mag. 124,000×.

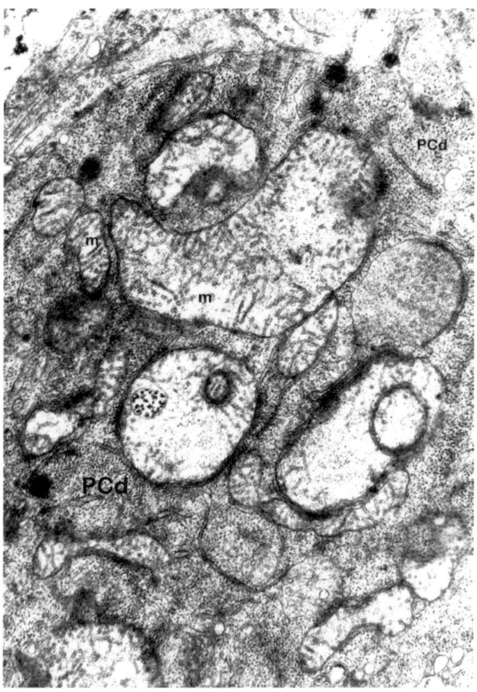

Figure 11.
Very large mitochondria (m) intermixed with small ones (m) in a dendritic profile of Purkinje cell (PCd) in the vermis of the cerebellum in a case of AD. Electron micrograph Mag. 124,000×.

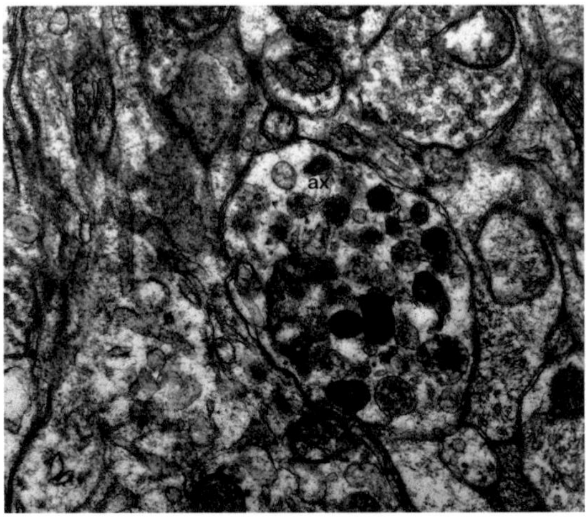

Figure 12.
Very small dense mitochondria in an axonic profile (ax) in the acoustic cortex in a case of AD. Electron micrograph Mag. 124,000×.

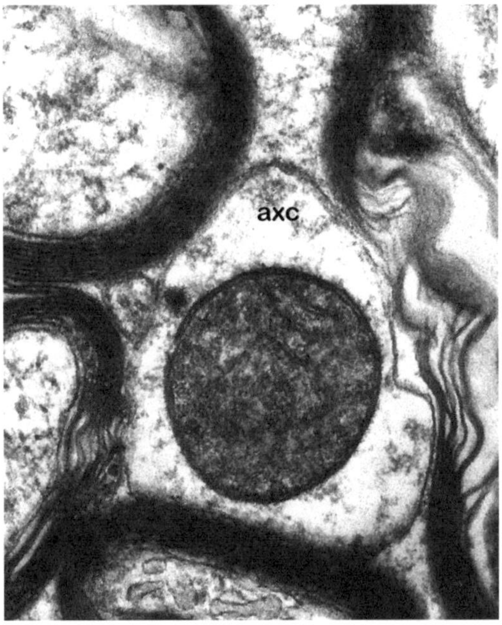

Figure 13.
Large mitochondrion in an axonic collateral among myelinated fibers in the prefrontal area of the cortex in a case of AD. Electron micrograph Mag. 124,000×.

morphological alterations of the synapses and dendritic spines coincide, as a rule, with marked mitochondrial alterations [22].

In morphometric estimation, the mitochondria in normal control aged brains appeared to have an average diameter of 250–650 nm and a mean axial ratio of 1.9 ± 0.2. The round or global mitochondria in normal controls appeared to have a mean mitochondrial radius of 350 nm. In Alzheimer's disease, ellipsoid mitochondria of Purkinje cells appeared to have an average diameter of 250–510 nm and a mean axial ratio of 1.7 ± 0.2. Round mitochondria were characterized by a mean radius of 280 nm.

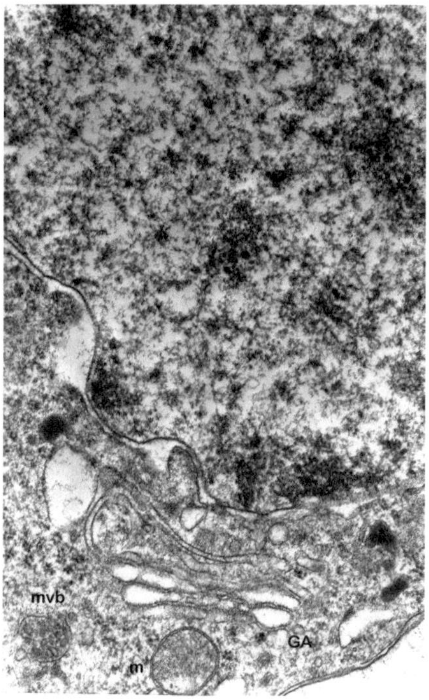

Figure 14.
Small mitochondrion (m) near dilated cisternae of Golgi apparatus (GA) and multivesicular body (mvb) in the soma of an astrocyte in the prefrontal area of the cortex of a case of AD. Electron micrograph Mag. 54,000×.

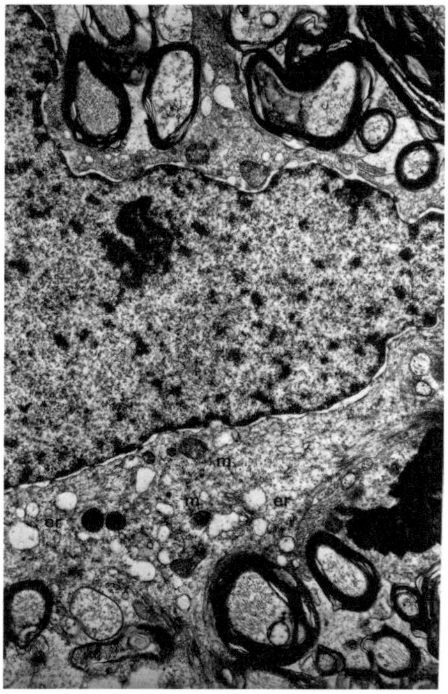

Figure 15.
Small mitochondria (m) among dilated cisternae of smooth endoplasmic reticulum (er) in the soma of an astrocyte in the parietal cortex of a case of AD. Electron micrograph Mag. 54,000×.

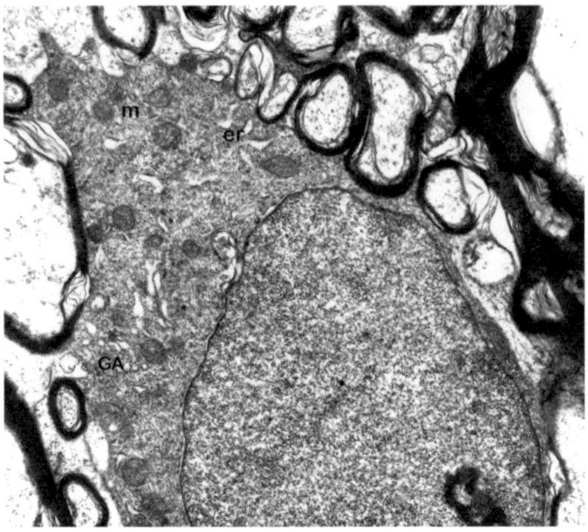

Figure 16.
Small mitochondria (m) among dilated cisternae of smooth endoplasmic reticulum (er) and fragmented cisternae of Golgi apparatus in the soma of an oligodendrocyte in the subcortical white matter of the parietal lobe of a case of AD. Electron micrograph Mag. 54,000×.

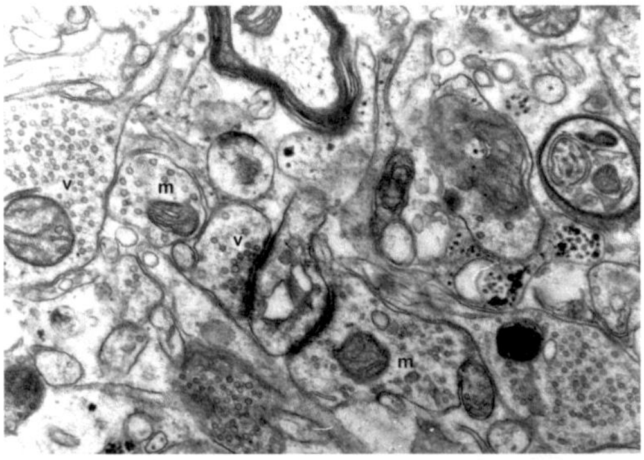

Figure 17.
Small mitochondria (m) in presynaptic profiles which show a dramatic poverty of synaptic vesicles (v) in the molecular layer of the cerebellum of AD. Electron micrograph Mag. 124,000×.

4. Discussion

Mitochondria play an essential role in energy supply of the cells, given that they provide most of the energy by oxidative phosphorylation of glucose, been basely key organelles for energy production involved in many metabolic pathways of the cell [98]. Mitochondrial dysfunction, associated with aging may be also a crucial factor in neurodegenerative disorders including Alzheimer's disease.

Decrease in energy metabolism and altered cytochrome C oxidase (CytOX) activity are among the earliest detectable defects in AD [99], affecting presumably neuronal plasticity and synaptogenesis. It is important to underline that reduced respiratory activity has also been reported in platelets of patients who suffered from AD [100], in the early stages of the disease. In addition, postmortem cytochrome-C oxidase activity is lower than normal in the cerebral cortex and in the platelets of AD patients [101] and mutations in cytochrome-C oxidase genes have been reported in late-onset AD [102].

Mitochondria and mtDNA are very sensitive to oxidative damage, such as protein oxidation and lipid peroxidation and inversely mitochondrial alterations may induce or enhance the existing oxidative stress, a fact pleading for an intimate and early association between oxidative stress and mitochondrial abnormalities [103, 104].

In addition, the combined effect of high calcium ions with oxidative stress may induce serious impairment of the mitochondrial function, leading to release of cytochrome C and triggering the initiation of the intrinsic pathway for apoptosis in many systems [105–107].

Oxidative stress can also enhance the production and the aggregation of Aβ [108] as well as the hyperphosphorylation of tau protein, which contribute extensively in the pathogenetic mechanism of AD [109]. The overproduction of Aβ peptide in AD induces fission and fragmentation of mitochondria, a fact that further increases oxidative stress and causes a considerable decline of energy production, which is associated with the increased expression of dynamin-related protein 1 (Drp1) [110]. The Aβ peptide enhances the activity of Drp1 protein in neurons, which subsequently induces morphological alteration of the mitochondria and increases the mitochondrial dysfunction in AD.

Mitochondrial alterations are closely connected with the over expression of the amyloid precursor protein (APP) and the amyloid-β peptide [58]. The Aβ peptides are generated either extracellularly or within the cisternae of the endoplasmic reticulum (ER) and the mitochondria. APP is folded and modified in the ER and transported through the Golgi complex to the plasma membrane. Transmembrane arrest of APP causes considerable impairment of mitochondrial function in neurons [111].

A substantial amount of amyloid-β peptide is generated in mitochondria-associated ER membranes (ER-MAMs or MAMs), which is a dynamic sub-compartment of the ER, which is connected with mitochondria [112]. In Alzheimer's disease, intraneuronal amyloid precursor protein and amyloid-β are mostly localized to mitochondria [112], where amyloid-β peptide may induce mitochondrial dysfunctions by interaction with cyclophilin D, which is a subunit of the mitochondrial permeability transition pore [113]. Amyloid-β peptide may also interact with Aβ binding alcohol dehydrogenase (ABAD) on the mitochondrial membranes and induce further mitochondrial dysfunction [114]. Moreover, alterations in the lipid composition of cellular membranes may influence proteolytic processing of AβPP and increase the release of Alzheimer's amyloid beta-peptide from membranes [115].

In addition, Aβ peptide inhibits protein influx in the mitochondria, resulting in mutation of mitochondrial DNA (mtDNA), aggravating therefore mitochondrial dysfunction and disintegration eventually [116]. Experimental studies, on the other hand, revealed that the soluble form of Aβ peptide causes a reduced mitochondrial membrane potential (MMP) and energy production [117].

Mitochondrial dysfunction on the other hand may play an important role for enhancing the neurotoxicity of the Aβ peptide in AD, aggravating furthermore the oxidative stress. Oxidative stress is reasonably associated with amyloid β peptide accumulation in the neocortex [118], a fact which plays a crucial role in the pathogenesis of Alzheimer's disease, inducing alterations to the cytoplasm of sensitive cells [119] by increasing reactive oxygen species (ROS) production [120]. This condition may cause further mitochondrial dysfunction, since the lack of histones in mitochondrial DNA makes them particularly vulnerable to oxidative stress [121, 122].

It is important that morphological alterations of the mitochondria in AD are observed in areas of the brain with minimal Alzheimer's pathology, such as in the cerebellum, the hypothalamus and the mammillary bodies [123] suggesting that they are independent of the accumulation of neurofibrillary tangles and neuritic plaques.

It is well known that shape and the size of the mitochondria are highly variable [124], since they undergo continual fission and fusion, which are necessary for cell survival and harmonious adaptation to changing conditions [125] and are related, at the same time, with the processes of biogenesis [126] and the mitophagy [127].

In addition, mitochondrial morphology is sometimes controlled by the cytoskeleton, namely the neurofilaments and the microtubules [128]. The change of the shape of the mitochondria occurs mostly during their course through axons, dendrites and synaptic terminals via anterograde transport [129].

Many proteins are also important for the mitochondrial morphological integrity and for binding to the cytoskeletal components [130]. Porin is a protein in the outer membrane of the mitochondria that forms voltage-dependent anionic channels, between the mitochondrial inter membrane space and the cytosol [131]. Porin may play crucial role in binding to cytoskeleton [132], because porin-rich domains mostly contain binding sites for MAP2. In addition, recent evidence suggest that amyloid β increases the contact points between endoplasmic reticulum and mitochondria, a phenomenon that occurs in cellular stress, which usually increases ER-mitochondrial coupling [133].

Normally, approximately one-third of the mitochondria are in motion along with microtubules and actin filaments [128, 134], transported to regions where energy requirement is particularly high. The number of the mitochondria is adjusted, according to the requirement of energy by the cell. It is reasonable that the dysfunctional mitochondria may undergo mitophagy [135], a fact which is associated with neurodegeneration [136] and many devastating conditions of the brain.

Morphometric studies of the mitochondria in non-nerve cells in AD revealed a significant reduction in mitochondrial density in endothelial cells [137] as well as in fibroblasts and other cells obtained from patients with AD [138]. Mitochondria from fibroblasts grown in tissue culture from skin samples taken during autopsy of patients of AD, took significantly less calcium than did mitochondria of fibroblasts from age matched normal controls, suggesting that Alzheimer's fibroblast mitochondria have impaired calcium transport processes and showed increased sensitivity to oxygenic free radicals [139].

The most dramatic morphological alterations of the mitochondria are seen in dendritic profiles and the synaptic terminals. The defective mitochondria in AD neurons may not supply adequate levels of adenosine triphosphate (ATP), which is very important factor at the synaptic level for normal neural communication. The low levels of cellular ATP at nerve terminals may lead to the loss of synapses and considerable decline of synaptic function, causing serious cognitive impairment and profound dementia ultimately.

Mitochondrial alterations in AD are observed also in astrocytes, although mitochondrial dynamics of astrocytes are not yet extensively studied. Astrocytes participate in the degradation of neuronal mitochondria via the process of transmitophagy [140] that occurs following internalization of axonal mitochondria by astrocytic processes, which normally contain very small mitochondria [141]. Astrocytic alterations have been described in cases of familial Alzheimer's disease [142] as well as in advanced cased of sporadic type of Alzheimer's disease [143], demonstrating evidence of the toxicity of the Aβ peptide [144]. The mitochondrial alterations of the astrocytes in early case of Alzheimer's disease enhance the noxious role of the Aβ peptide on the function and the integrity of the astrocytes [145] with serious implications on neuroprotection [146] due to the increased excitotoxicity, which would be a reasonable consequence of the disruption of glutamate/GABA-glutamine cycle [147].

In all of the cases, it was noticed that the morphological alterations of mitochondria in neurons and astrocytes are frequently associated with the fragmentation of Golgi apparatus and the decrease of the vesicles in cis- and trans-Golgi network [19, 56]. The morphological alterations of the mitochondria and the fragmentation of Golgi complex coincide with the dendritic and synaptic pathology in early cases of Alzheimer's disease [22, 148].

Understanding the important role the mitochondrial factor plays in the etiopathogenetic cascade of Alzheimer's disease [13], new therapeutic strategies aim at protecting the mitochondria [149] and preventing oxidative stress, calcium imbalance and eventual apoptosis might be beneficial in the treatment of early cases of AD.

5. Conclusions

The study in electron microscopy of various areas of the cerebral cortex, including the prefrontal area, the superior parietal lobe, the occipital pole, the visual cortex and the Hessl gyri of the temporal neocortex, and various areas of the cerebellar cortex, the hypothalamus, the mammillary bodies and the medial geniculate body in early cases of Alzheimer's disease, revealed serious morphological alterations of the mitochondria in the perikaryon, the dendritic branches the axons and the synapses.

The most dramatic alteration of the mitochondrial morphology was observed in the dendritic profiles, the dendritic spines and the synapses, associated with poverty of synaptic vesicles and accumulation of multi vesicular bodies.

The morphological alterations of the mitochondria were not dependent on the typical Alzheimer's pathology, since they were seen in areas with minimal β amyloid aggregations and no neurofibrillary tangles, such as the cerebellum, the hypothalamus and the visual cortex, suggesting that the mitochondrial alterations are not the direct consequence of amyloid toxicity.

Mitochondrial alterations were also seen in astrocytes and oligodendrocytes frequently in association with dilatation of the cisternae of the smooth endoplasmic reticulum and Golgi complex.

The mitochondria alterations induce a substantial decline of energy supply to neuronal processes, affecting the protein trafficking, the membrane dynamics as well as the synaptic activity, resulting in gradual synaptic and dendritic degeneration and in neuronal apoptosis eventually.

Mitochondria are strategic points in the pathogenetic field of Alzheimer's disease. New therapeutic strategies aiming at protecting the mitochondria, increasing the energy supply and preventing oxidative stress and calcium imbalance, might be beneficial in the treatment of early cases of AD.

Conflict of interest

No conflict of interest.

Nomenclature and abbreviations

AD Alzheimer's disease

Author details

Stavros J. Baloyannis[1,2]

1 Laboratory of Neuropathology and Electron Microscopy, Department of Neurology, Aristotelian University of Thessaloniki, Greece

2 Institute for Research on Alzheimer's Disease, Iraklion, Greece

*Address all correspondence to: sibh844@otenet.gr

References

[1] Reitz C, Mayeux R. Alzheimer disease: Epidemiology, diagnostic criteria, risk factors and biomarkers. Biochemical Pharmacology. 2014;**88**:640-651

[2] Cummings JL, Morstorf T, Zhong K. Alzheimer's disease drug-development pipeline: Few candidates, frequent failures. Alzheimer's Research & Therapy. 2014;**6**:37

[3] Schelke MW, Attia P, Palenchar D, Kaplan B, Mureb M, Ganzer CA, et al. Mechanisms of risk reduction in the clinical practice of Alzheimer's disease prevention. Frontiers in Aging Neuroscience. 2018;**10**:96

[4] Baloyannis SJ. Neuropathology of Dementia. Aristotelian University of Thessaloniki; 1993

[5] Alzheimer's Association. Alzheimer's disease facts and figures. Alzheimer's & Dementia. 2010;**6**:158-194

[6] Wisniewski HM, Wegiel J, Kotula L. Some neuropathological aspects of Alzheimer's disease and its relevance to other disciplines. Neuropathology and Applied Neurobiology. 1996;**22**:3-11

[7] Duyckaerts C, Delatour B, Potier MC. Classification and basic pathology of Alzheimer disease. Acta Neuropathologica. 2009;**118**:5-36

[8] Baloyannis S, Costa V, Arnaoutoglou A, Arnaoutoglou H. Synaptic alterations in the molecular layer of the cerebellum in Alzheimer's disease. Neuropathology and Applied Neurobiology. 1996;**22**:78-79

[9] Baloyannis SJ, Manolidis SL, Manolidis LS. Synaptic alterations in the vestibule-cerebellar system in Alzheimer's disease-a Golgi and electron microscope study. Acta Oto-Laryngologica. 2000;**120**:247-250

[10] Selkoe DJ. Alzheimer's disease is a synaptic failure. Science. 2002;**298**:789-791

[11] Poirel O, Mella S, Videau C, Ramet L, Davoli MA, Herzog E, et al. Moderate decline in select synaptic markers in the prefrontal cortex (BA9) of patients with Alzheimer's disease at various cognitive stages. Scientific Reports. 2018;**8**:938

[12] Baloyannis SJ, Costa V, Michmizos D. Mitochondrial alterations in Alzheimer's disease. American Journal of Alzheimer's Disease and Other Dementias. 2004;**19**:89-93

[13] Baloyannis SJ. Mitochondria: Strategic point in the field of Alzheimer's disease. Journal of Alzheimers and Neurodegenerative Diseases. 2016;**2**:004

[14] Iqbal K, Liu F, Gong CX, Grundke-Iqbal I. Tau in Alzheimer disease and related tauopathies. Current Alzheimer Research. 2010;**7**:656-664

[15] Mattson MP. Pathways towards and away from Alzheimer's disease. Nature. 2004;**430**:631-639

[16] Baloyannis SJ, Baloyannis IS. The vascular factor in Alzheimer's disease: A study in Golgi technique and electron microscopy. Journal of the Neurological Sciences. 2012;**322**:117-121

[17] Dickson DM. The pathogenesis of senile plaques. Journal of Neuropathology and Experimental Neurology. 1997;**56**:321-339

[18] Gandy S. The role of cerebral amyloid beta accumulation in common forms of Alzheimer disease. The Journal of Clinical Investigation. 2005;**115**:1121-1129

[19] Baloyannis S. The Golgi apparatus of Purkinje cells in Alzheimer's disease.

In: Bohl J, editor. Neuropathology Back to the Roots. Aachen, Germany: Shaker Vertag; 2002. pp. 1-10

[20] Hirai K, Aliev G, Nunomura A, et al. Mitochondrial abnormalities in Alzheimer's disease. The Journal of Neuroscience. 2001;**21**:3017-3023

[21] Baloyannis SJ, Baloyannis JS. Mitochondrial alterations in Alzheimer's disease. Neurobiology of Aging. 2004;**25**:405-406

[22] Baloyannis SJ. Mitochondria are related to synaptic pathology in Alzheimer's disease. International Journal of Alzheimer's Disease. 2011;**2011**:305395. DOI: 10.4061/2011/305395

[23] Cummings JL, Vinters HV, Cole GM, Khachaturian ZS. Alzheimer's disease etiologies, pathophysiology, cognitive reserve, and treatment opportunities. Neurology. 1998;**51**(1 Suppl 1):S2-S17

[24] Weinstein JD. Alzheimer's disease: Multiple causes requiring multiple therapies. Acta Scientific Medical Sciences. 2018;**2**:16-20

[25] Lendon CL, Ashall F, Goate AM. Exploring the etiology of Alzheimer disease using molecular genetics. Journal of the American Medical Association. 1997;**277**:825-831

[26] Breitner JC. Alzheimer's disease: Genetic theories of etiology. In: Handbook of Psychopharmacology. Boston, MA: Springer; 1988. pp. 207-235

[27] Selkoe DJ. Alzheimer's disease: Genes, proteins, and therapy. Physiological Reviews. 2001;**81**:741-766

[28] Mravec B, Horvathova L, Padova A. Brain under stress and Alzheimer's disease. Cellular and Molecular Neurobiology. 2018;**38**:73-84

[29] Rogers JO, Morrison JH. Quantitative morphology and regional and laminar distributions of senile plaques in Alzheimer's disease. The Journal of Neuroscience. 1985;**5**:2801-2808

[30] Sochocka M, Zwolinska K, Leszek J. The infectious etiology of Alzheimer's disease. Current Neuropharmacology. 2017;**15**:996-1009

[31] Jevtic S, Sengar AS, Salter MW, McLaurin J. The role of the immune system in Alzheimer disease: Etiology and treatment. Ageing Research Reviews. 2017;**40**:84-94

[32] Carlsen EM, Rasmussen R. Protein networks in Alzheimer's disease. Cell Systems. 2017;**4**:153-155

[33] Santos CY, Snyder PJ, Wu WC, Zhang M, Echeverria A, Alber J. Pathophysiologic relationship between Alzheimer's disease, cerebrovascular disease, and cardiovascular risk: A review and synthesis. Alzheimer's & Dementia: Diagnosis, Assessment & Disease Monitoring. 2017;**7**:69-87

[34] Ning K, Chen B, Sun F, Hobel Z, Zhao L, Matloff W, et al. Alzheimer's disease neuroimaging initiative. Classifying Alzheimer's disease with brain imaging and genetic data using a neural network framework. Neurobiology of Aging. 2018;**68**:151-158

[35] Bierer LM, Haroutunian V, Gabriel S, Knott PJ, Carlin LS, Purohit DP, et al. Neurochemical correlates of dementia severity in Alzheimer's disease: Relative importance of the cholinergic deficits. Journal of Neurochemistry. 1995;**64**:749-760

[36] Hampel H, Bürger K, Teipel SJ, Bokde AL, Zetterberg H, Blennow K. Core candidate neurochemical and imaging biomarkers of Alzheimer's disease. Alzheimer's & Dementia. 2008;**4**:38-48

[37] Atwood CS, Huang X, Moir RD, Tanzi RE, Bush AI. Role of free radicals

and metal ions in the pathogenesis of Alzheimer's disease. In: Metal Ions in Biological Systems. Abingdon-on-Thames. Routledge; 2018. pp. 309-364

[38] Murray HC, Swanson ME, Dieriks BV, Turner C, Faull RL, Curtis MA. Neurochemical characterization of PSA-NCAM+ cells in the human brain and phenotypic quantification in Alzheimer's disease entorhinal cortex. Neuroscience. 2018;**372**:289-303

[39] Musiek ES, Holtzman DM. Three dimensions of the amyloid hypothesis: Time, space and 'wingmen'. Nature Neuroscience. 2015;**18**:800

[40] Selkoe DJ, Hardy J. The amyloid hypothesis of Alzheimer's disease at 25 years. EMBO Molecular Medicine. 2016;**8**:595-608

[41] Manyevitch R, Protas M, Scarpiello S, Deliso M, Bass B, Nanajian A, et al. Evaluation of metabolic and synaptic dysfunction hypotheses of Alzheimer's disease (AD): A meta-analysis of CSF markers. Current Alzheimer Research. 2018;**15**:164-181

[42] Du X, Wang X, Geng M. Alzheimer's disease hypothesis and related therapies. Translational Neurodegeneration. 2018;7(2):1-7

[43] Kaufman SK, Del Tredici K, Thomas TL, Braak H, Diamond MI. Tau seeding activity begins in the transentorhinal/entorhinal regions and anticipates phospho-tau pathology in Alzheimer's disease and PART. Acta Neuropathologica. 2018;**136**:57-67

[44] Salinaro AT, Pennisi M, Di Paola R, Scuto M, Crupi R, Cambria MT, et al. Neuroinflammation and neurohormesis in the pathogenesis of Alzheimer's disease and Alzheimer-linked pathologies: Modulation by nutritional mushrooms. Immunity & Ageing. 2018;**15**:8

[45] Hampel H, Mesulam MM, Cuello AC, Farlow MR, Giacobini E, Grossberg GT, et al. The cholinergic system in the pathophysiology and treatment of Alzheimer's disease. Brain. 2018;**141**:1917-1933

[46] Vergallo A, Giampietri L, Baldacci F, Volpi L, Chico L, Pagni C, et al. Oxidative stress assessment in Alzheimer's disease: A clinic setting study. American Journal of Alzheimer's Disease and Other Dementias. 2018;**33**:35-41

[47] Baloyannis SJ. Brain capillaries in Alzheimer's disease. Hellenic Journal of Nuclear Medicine. 2015;**18**:152

[48] Di Marco LY, Venneri A, Farkas E, Evans PC, Marzo A, Frangi AF. Vascular dysfunction in the pathogenesis of Alzheimer's disease—A review of endothelium-mediated mechanisms and ensuing vicious circles. Neurobiology of Disease. 2015;**82**:593-606

[49] Daulatzai MA. Cerebral hypoperfusion and glucose hypometabolism: Key pathophysiological modulators promote neurodegeneration, cognitive impairment, and Alzheimer's disease. Journal of Neuroscience Research. 2017;**95**:943-972

[50] Le Page A, Dupuis G, Frost EH, Larbi A, Pawelec G, Witkowski JM, et al. Role of the peripheral innate immune system in the development of Alzheimer's disease. Experimental Gerontology. 2018;**107**:59-66

[51] Takeda S, Morishita R. Diabetes and Alzheimer's disease. In: Diabetes and Aging-related Complications. Singapore: Springer; 2018. pp. 101-111

[52] Folch J, Ettcheto M, Busquets O, Sánchez-López E, Castro-Torres R, Verdaguer E, et al. The implication of the brain insulin receptor in late onset Alzheimer's disease dementia. Pharmaceuticals. 2018;**11**:11. DOI: 10.3390/ph11010011

[53] Baloyannis SJ. Mitochondrial alterations in Alzheimer's disease. Journal of Alzheimer's Disease. 2006;**9**:119-126

[54] Swerdlow RH. Mitochondria and mitochondrial cascades in Alzheimer's disease. Journal of Alzheimer's Disease. 2018;**62**:1403-1416

[55] Stieber A, Mourelatos Z, Gonatas NK. In Alzheimer's disease the Golgi apparatus of a population of neurons without neurofibrillary tangles is fragmented and atrophic. The American Journal of Pathology. 1996;**148**:415-426

[56] Baloyannis SJ. Golgi apparatus and protein trafficking in Alzheimer's disease. Journal of Alzheimer's Disease. 2014;**42**:S153-S162

[57] Joshi G, Bekier MI, Wang Y. Golgi fragmentation in Alzheimer's disease. Frontiers in Neuroscience. 2015;**9**:340. DOI: 10.3389/fnins.2015.00340

[58] Cheignon C, Tomas M, Bonnefont-Rousselot D, Faller P, Hureau C, Collin F. Oxidative stress and the amyloid beta peptide in Alzheimer's disease. Redox Biology. 2018;**14**:450-464

[59] Džinić T, Dencher NA. Oxygen concentration and oxidative stress modulate the influence of Alzheimer's disease Aβ1-42 peptide on human cells. Oxidative Medicine and Cellular Longevity. 2018;**2018**:16. DOI: 10.1155/2018/7567959. Article ID: 7567959

[60] Kametani F, Hasegawa M. Reconsideration of amyloid hypothesis and tau hypothesis in Alzheimer's disease. Frontiers in Neuroscience. 2018;**12**:25. DOI: 10.3389/fnins.2018.00025

[61] Wang X, Wang W, Li L, Perry G, Lee HG, Zhu X. Oxidative stress and mitochondrial dysfunction in Alzheimer's disease. Biochimica et Biophysica Acta (BBA)-Molecular Basis of Disease. 2014;**1842**:1240-1247

[62] Atamna H, Frey WH II. Mechanisms of mitochondrial dysfunction and energy deficiency in Alzheimer's disease. Mitochondrion. 2007;7:297-310

[63] Du H, Guo L, Yan SS. Synaptic mitochondrial pathology in Alzheimer's disease. Antioxidants and Redox Signaling. 2012;**16**:1467-1475

[64] Bennett RE, Robbins AB, Hu M, Cao X, Betensky RA, Clark T, et al. Tau induces blood vessel abnormalities and angiogenesis-related gene expression in P301L transgenic mice and human Alzheimer's disease. Proceedings of the National Academy of Sciences. 2018;**115**:E1289-E1298

[65] Polverino A, Grimaldi M, Sorrentino P, Jacini F, D'Ursi AM, Sorrentino G. Effects of acetylcholine on β-amyloid-induced cPLA2 activation in the TB neuroectodermal cell line: Implications for the pathogenesis of Alzheimer's disease. Cellular and Molecular Neurobiology. 2018;**38**:817-826

[66] Iaccarino L, Tammewar G, Ayakta N, Baker SL, Bejanin A, Boxer AL, et al. Local and distant relationships between amyloid, tau and neurodegeneration in Alzheimer's disease. NeuroImage: Clinical. 2018;**17**:452-464

[67] Saraiva AA, Borges MM, Madeira MD, Tavares MA, Paula-Barbosa MM. Mitochondrial abnormalities in cortical dendrites from patients with Alzheimer's disease. Journal of Submicroscopic Cytology. 1985;**17**:459-464

[68] Li Z, Okamoto KI, Hayashi Y, Sheng M. The importance of dendritic mitochondria in the morphogenesis and plasticity of spines and synapses. Cell. 2004;**119**:873-887

[69] Baloyannis SJ. Dendritic pathology in Alzheimer's disease. Journal of the Neurological Sciences. 2009;**283**:153-157

[70] McGeer EG, McGeer PL. Innate immunity in Alzheimer's disease. Molecular Interventions. 2001;**1**:22-29

[71] McGeer PL, McGeer EG. Inflammation, autotoxicity and Alzheimer disease. Neurobiology of Aging. 2001;**22**:799-809

[72] Boza-Serrano A, Yang Y, Paulus A, Deierborg T. Innate immune alterations are elicited in microglial cells before plaque deposition in the Alzheimer's disease mouse model 5xFAD. Scientific Reports. 2018;**8**:1550

[73] Kunkle BW, Grenier-Boley B, Sims R, Bis JC, Naj AC, Boland A, et al. Meta-analysis of genetic association with diagnosed Alzheimer's disease identifies novel risk loci and implicates Abeta, Tau, immunity and lipid processing. bioRxiv. 2018:294629

[74] Lewis MR, Lewis WH. Mitochondria in tissue culture. Science. 1914;**39**:330-333

[75] Harman D. The biologic clock: The mitochondria? Journal of the American Geriatrics Society. 1972;**20**:145-147

[76] Lopez-Otin C, Blasco MA, Partridge L, Serrano M, Kroemer G. The hallmarks of aging. Cell. 2013;**153**:1194-1217

[77] Hughes BG, Hekimi S. A mild impairment of mitochondrial electron transport has sex-specific effects on lifespan and aging in mice. PLoS One. 2011;**6**:e26116

[78] Beal M, Hyman B, Koroshetz W. Do defects in mitochondrial energy metabolism underlie the pathology of neurodegenerative diseases? Trends in Neurosciences. 1993;**16**:125-131

[79] Mentzies F, Cookson M, Taylor R, et al. Mitochondrial dysfunction in a cell culture model of familial amyotrophic lateral sclerosis. Brain. 2002;**125**:1522-1533

[80] Perry G, Nunomura A, Hirai K, Takeda A, Aliev G, Smith M. Oxidative damage in Alzheimer's disease: The metabolic dimention. International Journal of Developmental Neuroscience. 2000;**18**:417-421

[81] Edland SD, Silverman JM, Peskind ER, Tsuang D, Wijsman E, Morris JC. Increased risk of dementia in mothers of Alzheimer's disease cases: Evidence for maternal inheritance. Neurology. 1996;**47**:254-256

[82] Bassett SS, Avramopoulos D, Fallin D. Evidence for parent of origin effect in late- onset Alzheimer disease. American Journal of Medical Genetics. 2002;**114**:679-686

[83] Debette S, Wolf PA, Beiser A, Au R, Himali JJ, Pikula A, et al. Association of parental dementia with cognitive and brain MRI measures in middle-aged adults. Neurology. 2009;**73**:2071-2078

[84] Morris JC, Heyman A, Mohs RC, Hughes JP, Van Belle G, Fillenbaum GD, et al. The consortium to establish a registry for Alzheimer's disease (CERAD): I. Clinical and neuropsychological assessment of Alzheimer's disease. Neurology. 1989;**39**:1159-1165

[85] Dubois B, Feldman HH, Jacova C, DeKosky ST, Barberger-Gateau P, Cummings J, et al. Research criteria for the diagnosis of Alzheimer's disease: Revising the NINCDS-ADRDA criteria. The Lancet Neurology. 2007;**6**:734-746

[86] McKhann GM, Knopman DS, Chertkow H, Hyman BT, Jack CR Jr, Kawas CH, et al. The diagnosis of dementia due to Alzheimer's disease: Recommendations from

the National Institute on Aging-Alzheimer's Association workgroups on diagnostic guidelines for Alzheimer's disease. Alzheimer's & Dementia. 2011;7:263-269

[87] Schindler SE, Jasielec MS, Weng H, Hassenstab JJ, Grober E, McCue LM, et al. Neuropsychological measures that detect early impairment and decline in preclinical Alzheimer disease. Neurobiology of Aging. 2017;**56**:25-32

[88] Tombaugh TN, McIntyre NJ. The mini-mental state examination: A comprehensive review. Journal of the American Geriatrics Society. 1992;**40**:922-935

[89] Arevalo-Rodriguez I, Smailagic N, I Figuls MR, Ciapponi A, Sanchez-Perez E, Giannakou A, et al. Mini-mental state examination (MMSE) for the detection of Alzheimer's disease and other dementias in people with mild cognitive impairment (MCI). Cochrane Database of Systematic Reviews. 2015;**5**(3):CD010783

[90] Mattis S. Dementia Rating Scale Professional Manual, Psychological Assessment Resources; Odessa, Fla, USA; 1988

[91] Dean PM, Cerhan JH. Correction for a potentially biased item on the mattis dementia rating scale. American Journal of Alzheimer's Disease and Other Dementias. 2013;**28**:734-737. DOI: 10.1177/1533317513504610

[92] Rosen WG, Mohs RC, Davis KL. A new rating scale for Alzheimer's disease. The American Journal of Psychiatry. 1984;**141**:1356-1364

[93] Harrison JC, Minassian SL, Jenkins L, et al. A neuropsychological test battery for use in Alzheimer disease clinical trials. Archives of Neurology. 2007;**64**:1323-1329

[94] Hollocks MJ, Brookes RL, Morris RG, Markus HS. The Brief Memory and Executive Test (BMET): A cognitive screening tool to detect and differentiate vascular cognitive impairment and Alzheimer's disease. International Journal of Geriatric Psychiatry. 2018;**33**:e273-e279

[95] Kogure D, Matsuda H, Ohnishi T, Asada T, Uno M, Kunihiro T, et al. Longitudinal evaluation of early Alzheimer's disease using brain perfusion SPECT. Journal of Nuclear Medicine. 2000;**41**:1155-1162

[96] Sotelo C, Hillman DE, Zamora AJ, Llinás R. Climbing fiber deafferentation: Its action on Purkinje cell dendritic spines. Brain Research. 1975;**98**:574-581

[97] Baloyannis SJ, Mavroudis I, Mitilineos D, Baloyannis IS, Costa VG. The hypothalamus in Alzheimer's disease: A Golgi and electron microscope study. American Journal of Alzheimer's Disease and Other Dementias. 2015;**30**:478-487

[98] Beal MF. Aging, energy, and oxidative stress in neurodegenerative diseases. Annals of Neurology. 1995;**38**:357-366

[99] Cardoso S, Proenca M, Santos S, Santana I, Oliveira C. Cytochrome c oxidase is decreased in Alzheimer's disease platelets. Neurobiology of Aging. 2004;**25**:105-110

[100] Fisar Z, Hroudová J, Hansíková H, Lelková P, Wenchich L, Jirák R, et al. Mitochondrial respiration in the platelets of patients with Alzheimer's disease. Current Alzheimer Research. 2016;**13**:930-941

[101] Mutisaya EM, Bowling AC, Beal MF. Cortical cytochrome oxidase activity is reduced in Alzheimer's disease. Journal of Neurochemistry. 1994;**63**:2179-2184

[102] Davis RE, Miller S, Herrnstadt C, et al. Mutations in mitochondrial

cytochrome c oxidase genes segregate with late-onset Alzheimer disease. Proceedings of the National Academy of Sciences of the United States of America. 1997;**94**:4526-4531

[103] Federico A, Cardaioli E, Da Pozzo P, Formichi P, Gallus GN, Radi E. Mitochondria, oxidative stress and neurodegeneration. Journal of the Neurological Sciences. 2012;**322**:254-262

[104] Mancuso M, Coppede F, Migliore L, Siciliano G, Murri L. Mitochondrial dysfunction, oxidative stress and neurodegeneration. Journal of Alzheimer's Disease. 2006;**10**:59-73

[105] Radi E, Formichi P, Battisti C, Federico A. Apoptosis and oxidative stress in neurodegenerative diseases. Journal of Alzheimer's Disease. 2014;**42**(Suppl 3):S125-S152

[106] Butterfield DA. The 2013 SFRBM discovery award: Selected discoveries from the butterfield laboratory of oxidative stress and its sequela in brain in cognitive disorders exemplified by Alzheimer disease and chemotherapy induced cognitive impairment. Free Radical Biology & Medicine. 2014;**74**:157-174

[107] Hamanaka RB, Chandel NS. Mitochondrial reactive oxygen species regulate cellular signaling and dictate biological outcomes. Trends in Biochemical Sciences. 2010;**35**:505-513

[108] Zhao Y, Zhao B. Oxidative stress and the pathogenesis of Alzheimer's disease. Oxidative Medicine and Cellular Longevity. 2013;**2013**:316523

[109] Alonso AD, Grundke-Iqbal I, Iqbal K. Alzheimer's disease hyperphosphorylated tau sequesters normal tau into tangles of filaments and disassembles microtubules. Nature Medicine. 1996;**2**:783-787

[110] Cho DH, Nakamura T, Fang J, Cieplak P, Godzik A, Gu Z, et al. S-Nitrosylation of Drp 1 mediates beta-amyloid-related mitochondrial fission and neuronal injury. Science. 2009;**324**:102-105

[111] Anandatheerthavarada HK, Biswas G, Robin M-A, Avadhani NG. Mitochondrial targeting and a novel transmembrane arrest of Alzheimer's amyloid precursor protein impairs mitochondrial function in neuronal cells. The Journal of Cell Biology. 2003;**161**:41-54

[112] De Strooper B, Scorrano L. Close encounter: Mitochondria, endoplasmic reticulum and Alzheimer's disease. The EMBO Journal. 2012;**31**:4095-4097

[113] Du H, Guo L, Fang F, et al. Cyclophilin D deficiency attenuates mitochondrial and neuronal perturbation and ameliorates learning and memory in Alzheimer's disease. Nature Medicine. 2008;**14**:1097-1105

[114] Lustbader JW, Cirilli M, Lin C, Xu HW, Takuma K, Wang N, et al. ABAD directly links Aβ to mitochondrial toxicity in Alzheimer's disease. Science. 2004;**304**:448-452

[115] Lemkul JA, Bevan DR. Lipid composition influences the release of Alzheimer's amyloid beta-peptide from membranes. Protein Science. 2011;**20**:1530-1545

[116] Lakatos A, Derbeneva O, Younes D, Keator D, Bakken T, Lvova M, et al. Association between mitochondrial DNA variations and Alzheimer's disease in the ADNI cohort. Neurobiology of Aging. 2010;**31**:1355-1363

[117] Rhein V, Song X, Wiesner A, Ittner LM, Baysang G, Meier F, et al. Amyloid-β and tau synergistically impair the oxidative phosphorylation system in triple transgenic Alzheimer's disease mice. Proceedings of the

National Academy of Sciences of the United States of America. 2009;**106**:20057-20062

[118] Morais Cardoso S, Swerdlow R, Oliveira C. Induction of cytochrome c-mediated apoptosis by amyloid beta 25-35 requires functional mitochondria. Brain Research. 2002;**931**:117-125

[119] Lustbader J, Cirilli M, Lin C, et al. ABAD directly links Abeta to mitochondrial toxicity in Alzheimer's disease. Science. 2004;**304**:448-453

[120] Sheehan J, Swerdlow R, Miller S, et al. Calcium homeostasis and reactive oxygen species production in cells transformed by mitochondria from individuals with sporadic Alzheimer's disease. The Journal of Neuroscience. 1997;**17**:4612-4622

[121] Mecocci P, MacGarvey U, Beal MF. Oxidative damage to mitochondrial DNA is increased in Alzheimer's disease. Annals of Neurology. 1994;**36**:747-751

[122] Wang J, Xiong S, Xie C, et al. Increased oxidative damage in nuclear and mitochondrial DNA in Alzheimer's disease. Journal of Neurochemistry. 2005;**93**:953-962

[123] Baloyannis SJ, Mavroudis I, Baloyannis IS, Costa VG. Mammillary bodies in Alzheimer's disease: A Golgi and electron microscope study. American Journal of Alzheimer's Disease and Other Dementias. 2016;**31**:247-256

[124] Bereiter-Hahn J, Vöth M. Dynamics of mitochondria in living cells: Shape changes, dislocations, fusion, and fission of mitochondria. Microscopy Research and Technique. 1994;**27**:198-219

[125] Youle RJ, van der Bliek AM. Mitochondrial fission, fusion and stress. Science. 2012;**337**:1062-1065

[126] Onyango IG, Lu J, Rodova M, Lezi E, Crafter AB, Swerdlow RH. Regulation of neuron mitochondrial biogenesis and relevance to brain health. Biochimica et Biophysica Acta. 2010;**1802**:228-234

[127] Kim I, Rodriguez-Enriquez S, Lemasters JJ. Selective degradation of mitochondria by mitophagy. Archives of Biochemistry and Biophysics. 2007;**462**:245-253

[128] Leterrier JF, Rusakov DA, Nelson BD, Linden M. Interactions between brain mitochondria and cytoskeleton: Evidence for specialized outer membrane domains involved in the association of cytoskeleton-associated proteins to mitochondria in situ and in vitro. Microscopy Research and Technique. 1994;**27**:233-261

[129] Hollenbeck PJ, Saxton WM. The axonal transport of mitochondria. Journal of Cell Science. 2005;**118**: 5411-5419

[130] Truscott K, Pfanner N, Voos W. Transport of proteins into mitochondria. Reviews of Physiology, Biochemistry and Pharmacology. 2001;**143**:81-136

[131] Lauterwasser J, Todt F, Zerbes RM, Nguyen TN, Craigen W, Lazarou M, et al. The porin VDAC2 is the mitochondrial platform for Bax retrotranslocation. Scientific Reports. 2016;**6**:32994

[132] Wagner O, Lifshitz J, Janmey P, et al. Mechanisms of mitochondria-neurofilament interactions. The Journal of Neuroscience. 2003;**23**:9046-9058

[133] Bravo R, Vicencio JM, Parra V, et al. Increased ER-mitochondrial coupling promotes mitochondrial respiration and bioenergetics during early phases of ER stress. Journal of Cell Science. 2011;**124**:2143-2152

[134] Schwarz TL. Mitochondrial trafficking in neurons. Cold Spring

Harbor Perspectives in Biology. 2013;**5**(6)

[135] Scherz-Shouval R, Elazar Z. Regulation of autophagy by ROS: Physiology and pathology. Trends in Biochemical Sciences. 2011;**36**:30-38

[136] Karbowski M, Neutzner A. Neurodegeneration as a consequence of failed mitochondrial maintenance. Acta Neuropathologica. 2012;**123**: 157-171

[137] Stewart P, Hayakawa K, Akers M, Vinters H. A morphometric study of the blood-brain barrier in Alzheimer's disease. Laboratory Investigation. 1992;**67**:734-742

[138] Blass J, Fheu R, Gibson G. Inheritent abnormalities in energy metabolism in Alzheimer's disease: Interaction with cerebrovascular compromise. Annals of the New York Academy of Sciences. 2000;**903**:204-221

[139] Peterson C, Golman JE. Alterations in calcium content and biochemical processes in cultured skin fibroblasts from aged and Alzheimer donors. Proceedings of the National Academy of Sciences of the United States of America. 1986;**83**:2758-2762

[140] Davis CH, Kim KY, Bushong EA, et al. Transcellular degradation of axonal mitochondria. Proceedings of the National Academy of Sciences of the United States of America. 2014;**111**(26):9633-9638

[141] Derouiche A, Haseleu J, Korf HW. Fine astrocyte processes contain very small mitochondria: Glial oxidative capability may fuel transmitter metabolism. Neurochemical Research. 2015;**40**(12):2402-2413

[142] Rodríguez-Arellano JJ, Parpura V, Zorec R, et al. Astrocytes in physiological aging and Alzheimer's disease. Neuroscience. 2016;**323**:170-182

[143] Osborn LM, Kamphuis W, Wadman WJ, et al. Astrogliosis: An integral player in the pathogenesis of Alzheimer's disease. Progress in Neurobiology. 2016;**144**:121-141

[144] Abramov AY, Canevari L, Duchen MR. Beta-amyloid peptides induce mitochondrial dysfunction and oxidative stress in astrocytes and death of neurons through activation of NADPH oxidase. Journal of Neuroscience. 2004;**24**(2):565-575

[145] Pagani L, Eckert A. Amyloid-Beta interaction with mitochondria. International Journal of Alzheimer's Disease. 2011;**2011**:925050

[146] Voloboueva LA, Suh SW, Swanson RA, et al. Inhibition of mitochondrial function in astrocytes: Implications for neuroprotection. Journal of Neurochemistry. 2007;**102**(4):1383-1394

[147] Bak LK, Schousboe A, Waagepetersen HS. The glutamate/GABA-glutamine cycle: Aspects of transport, neurotransmitter homeostasis and ammonia transfer. Journal of Neurochemistry. 2006;**98**(3):641-653

[148] Nakamura T, Lipton SA. Redox modulation by S-nitrosylation contributes to protein misfolding, mitochondrial dynamics, and neuronal synaptic damage in neurodegenerative diseases. Cell Death and Differentiation. 2011;**18**:1478-1486

[149] Singh N, Ghosh KK. Recent advances in the antioxidant therapies for Alzheimer's Disease: Emphasis on natural antioxidants. In: Pathology, Prevention and Therapeutics of Neurodegenerative Disease. Singapore: Springer; 2019. pp. 253-263

Chapter 4

Putative Involvement of Thiol Protease Inhibitor in the Function of Alzheimer Drug

Fakhra Amin and Bilqees Bano

Abstract

The intermolecular structure gets altered when drug-protein interaction takes place. It brings about alterations in the conformation of protein. An acetyl cholinesterase inhibitor (AChE) is the most used drug for patients who are suffering from Alzheimer's disease to curb its instigated symptoms. So, it is used as first-line defense in the insightful symptoms. This study is of concern with the interaction of cystatin purified from buffalo brain with its simple tri-step procedure including alkaline action, ammonium sulfate fractionation, and gel filtration chromatography on Sephadex G-75 with % yield of 64.13 and fold purification of 384.7. The inhibitor (brain cystatin (BC)) showed a single papain inhibitory peak drifted as single band on native PAGE; this purified inhibitor was interacted with donepezil to analyze the side effect of this drug since cystatin is an important regulatory protein that maintains the protease antiprotease balance. The conformational change was predicted when the UV spectra of cystatin was analyzed in the presence of donepezil contextual with the fluorescence spectra, but the fluorescence spectra showed 40 nm of red shift suggesting the change on interaction leading to a conclusion that donepezil is pertinent to imbalance to protease and antiprotease inhibitor perhaps the side effect of drug.

Keywords: acetyl cholinesterase (ach), acetyl cholinesterase inhibitor (AChE), Alzheimer's disease (AD), brain cystatin, (BC), thiol protease inhibitor

1. Introduction

Brain is exposed to a variety of neuromodulating agents given as therapy. The consequential action of these agents should be investigated to have the knowledge of their side influence. The primary degenerative disease of brain is dementia subsequently causing Alzheimer's disease. It is instigated in late life with cumulative properties like diminishing of memory, cognition, linguistic ability, and judgment. It is an advanced brain disorder relating to a person's inability to learn, reason, and carry out daily activities [1, 2]. The significant neurotransmitter acetylcholine is associated with normal functioning of the brain, and if the level of acetylcholine goes down in the cerebral cortex, this promulgates to Alzheimer's disease, the debilitating brain condition [3, 4].

Alzheimer's disease (AD) patients have lesser level of acetylcholine with the progressive abnormalities in cholinergic neurons. One line of attack to reduce the impact of these abnormalities is to obstruct the relevant enzyme AChE (acetylcholinesterase) which acts as a foremost agent in the breakdown of acetylcholine (ACh) [2]. Acetylcholine hydrolysis into choline and acetate is prevented by AChE inhibitors in the synaptic clefts and ensuing in activating cholinergic transmission [3]. Donepezil (**Figure 1**) is a piperidine-class *(piperidine is a widely used building block and chemical reagent in the synthesis of organic compounds, including pharmaceuticals; piperidine is a widely used secondary amine)* AChE inhibitor, sensibly designed especially for Alzheimer's disease [5, 6]. It is used to improve cognitive function in patients of AD and shows no sign of hepatotoxicity [7–9]. The trade name of this drug is Aricept and it functions as an acetylcholinesterase inhibitor [10]. It has 100% of an oral bioavailability and easily passes the blood–brain barrier. Shows the half life of 70 hrs. The primary action of donepezil is by plummeting the breakdown of acetylcholine thus amassing the concentration of acetylcholine in the brain retaining back to its normal function [11].

The major neuropathological hallmarks of AD are senile plaque, neurofibrillary tangles, and neuronal loss. Both cathepsins and cystatins (cystatin A and B) are found in close association with senile plague, cerebrovascular amyloid deposits, and neurofibrillary tangles in Alzheimer's disease, Parkinson's, and patients suffering from senile dementia supporting the fact that they are amyloid constituents. Recent researches have shown that cathepsins are one of the most important proteases involved in the processing of neuropeptides in the central nervous system (CNS) of brain (**Figure 2**) [12], while cystatin C is also existing in high concentration and their concentration relevant in brain diseases. Cysteine proteinases in normal persons help in β-peptide clearing. The disturbance between the accumulative action of cathepsins and cystatins may lead to aggregation of potentially amyloidogenic fragment collection aggravates to form amyloid fibrils in nerve cells of AD patients causing cystatin concentration to shrink (**Figure 3**). Generated by imbalance of cathepsins and cystatin, these potentially amyloidogenic fragments at liberty into the extracellular space cause the aggravation of disease [12].

The powerful regulatory system is constituted by cystatins for endogenous cysteine proteinases (cathepsins) which are often permeable from the lysosomes of dying or diseased cells [13]. Cystatins are the natural inhibitors of cysteine proteases with wide occurrence in tissues and cells which belong to a super family of proteins [14]. Cystatin super family has been divided into three families on the basis of homology, inhibition of target enzymes, and presence or absence of disulfide bonds.

Family 1, also called as stefins, includes members of low-molecular-weight proteins (11 kDa) which lack disulfide bonds and carbohydrate contents. This family includes cystatins A and B and stefins C and D.

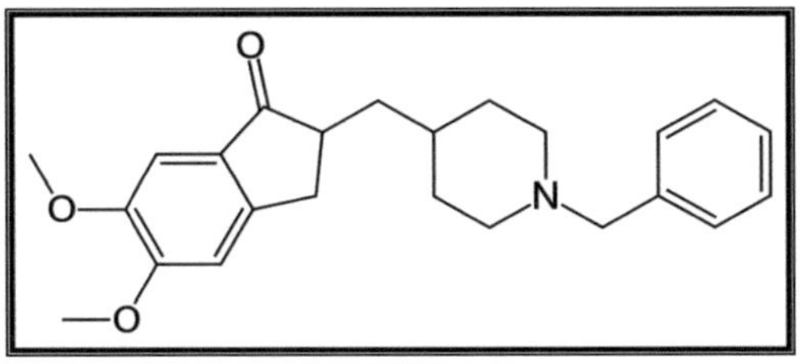

Figure 1.
Structure of donepezil [17].

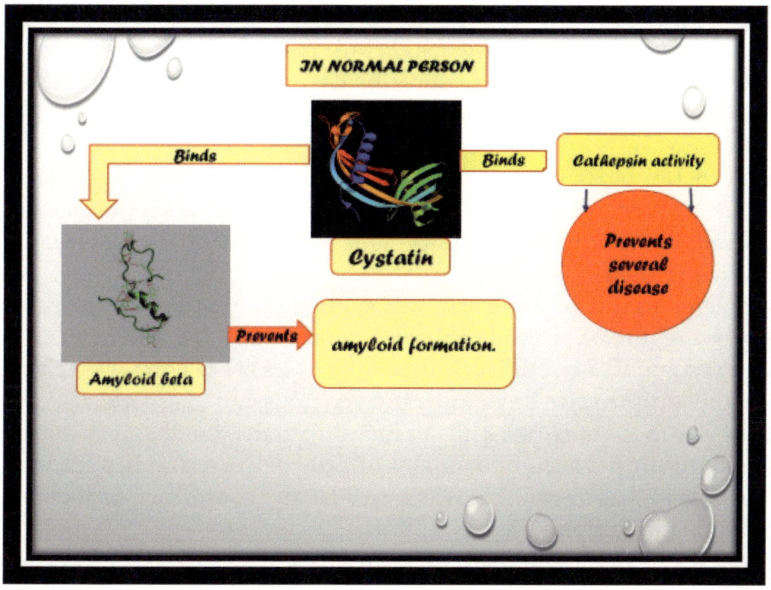

Figure 2.
Graphical abstract – Showing the function of cystatin in brain, how it is combating the several diseases.

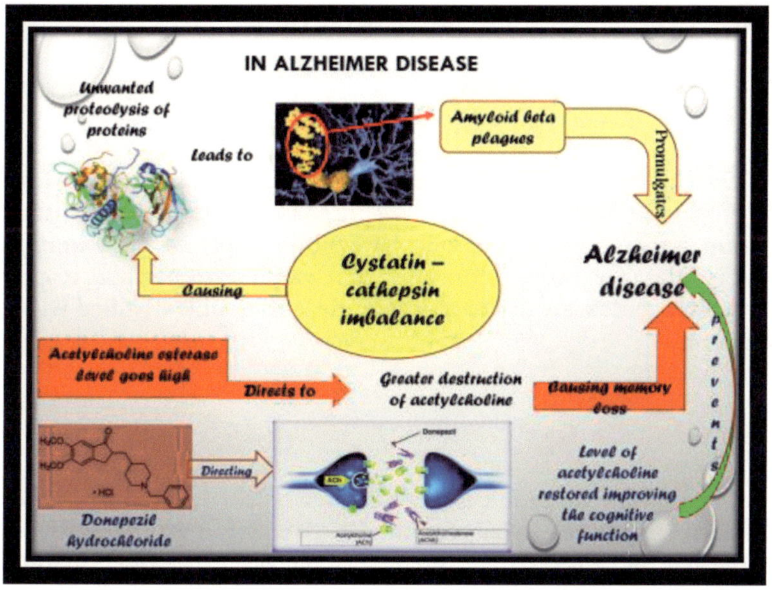

Figure 3.
Graphical abstract-2.

The figure shows the detailed interaction of cystatin-cathepsin imbalance and the role of acetylcholine esterase inhibitor as function in restoration of Alzheimer's diseases. They are found both in the body fluids and cells. Common illustration is cystatin C.

Kininogens or family 3 cystatins are large precursor molecules of the vasoactive kinins. They are glycoproteins of single chain that perform the multiple biological functions such as kinin delivery, induction of endogenous blood coagulation cascade, and acute phase response intercession. They are inhabitants of blood plasma [15].

Cystatins tightly bind and impede the activity of cathepsins; if the activity of cathepsins is not regulated, it instigates chronic diseases [13]. Senile plaque, cerebrovascular amyloid deposits, and neurofibrillary tangles in Alzheimer's disease are all the ramifications of imbalance between proteinases and their endogenous inhibitor cystatins [1].

Normal functioning of the brain is balanced by maintaining the level of acetylcholine and acetylcholinesterase inhibitor [16]. A previous report showed that donepezil binds along with HSA modifying it conformationally by effecting its free concentration in plasma [17].

The supplementation of donepezil was explored to find out any effect on cystatin (major regulator of thiol proteases: cathepsins B, H, and L, etc.) in the mammalian system. If the activity of these proteases is not controlled, it will lead to protease and antiprotease imbalance and repercussion to several diseases [18]. Therefore, it was thought worthwhile to investigate the donepezil cystatin binding and its role in the proper accomplishment of drug delivery and if it lead to kind of side effects as well as to gain knowledge about any conformational change in cystatin effecting its activity?

The study shows that the imbalance of protease-antiprotease purportedly leads the way to Alzheimer's disease, while the presence of drug donepezil unfolds cystatin which becomes unfit to bind cathepsins leading to a number of diseases as a considerable side effect of the drug. As cystatins play significant role in several diseases like, cancer and cardiovascular diseases [19]. Therefore, the usage of donepezil in such patients requires additional attention.

2. Materials

Papain (99% purity) was obtained from Sigma Chemical Company (St. Louis, USA). Donepezil (an Alzheimer drug) was purchased from Ranbaxy (India). The solutions were prepared in 50 mM phosphate buffer of pH 7.4. Salts were purchased from Merck (India). The protein concentration was determined spectrophotometrically. All other reagents were of analytical grade, and double distilled water was used throughout.

3. Methods

Purification of brain cystatins. Buffalo brain whole mass (150 g) was brought fresh from slaughter house in a box containing ice packs. It was carefully washed and rinsed with water, eliminating thin membrane and nerves by forceps, and the whole brain tissue was homogenized in 50 mM sodium phosphate buffer (300 mL) of pH 7.5 containing 0.15 M NaCl, 3 mM EDTA, and 2% n-butanol. After centrifugation at 11,000 rpm for 15 min at 40°C, residue was cast off, and the supernatant was further processed. The procedure involved a combination of alkaline treatment (pH 11.0), ammonium sulfate fractionation, and gel filtration chromatography. The brain was homogenized and fractionated with ammonium sulfate between 40 and 60% saturation; the precipitated protein was then dialyzed against 50 mM sodium phosphate buffer pH 7.4 containing 0.1 M NaCl. Elution profile showed two protein peaks—one major and one minor called as peak-I and peak-II. Peak-I is conforming to high-molecular-weight buffalo brain cystatin with significant inhibitory activity and protein content; however, peak-II with insignificant protein concentration and low inhibitory activity was not taken into consideration for further studies. Peak-I named as BC was purified with fold purification of 384.72 and yield of 64.13%.

Papain inhibitory fractions of peak-I were pooled, concentrated, and checked for purity. Five milliliter fractions were collected and assayed for protein and cystatin activity. Homogeneity of the preparation was investigated by 7.5% PAGE [20].

4. Spectroscopic studies

4.1 Fluorescence spectra of brain cystatin with drug

Brain cystatin (BC) (1 μM) was incubated for 30 min with subsequent higher concentration of donepezil in 0.05 M sodium phosphate buffer pH 7.5 in a final reaction volume of 1 mL at room temperature. The same buffer is used for preparation of drug solutions. Fluorescence measurements were carried out on a Shimadzu Spectroflourimeter model RF-5301PC (Shimadzu, Japan) equipped with a 150 W Xenon lamp and a slit width of 10 nm at 298 K. The fluorescence was recorded in wavelength region 300–400 nm after exciting the protein at 280 nm. The slits were set at 10 nm for excitation and emission. The path length of the sample was 1 cm.

4.2 UV spectra of cystatin in the presence of donepezil

The UV measurement of brain cystatin in the presence and absence of drug was made in the range of 200–300 nm, and the inhibitor (cystatin) concentration was fixed at 1 μM, while the drug concentration was varied from 0.16 to 1.6 μM. Absorption spectra were recorded on a double-beam Shimadzu UV-vis spectrophotometer UV-1700 using a cuvette of 1 cm path length.

4.3 Activity measurement of brain cystatin in the presence of donepezil

The inhibitory activity of the purified inhibitor (BC) under native conditions was assessed by its ability to inhibit caseinolytic activity of papain by the method of Kunitz [21]. The inhibitor (1 μM) was incubated with increasing concentrations of donepezil at 25°C for 30 min before the activity was measured. Activity of untreated BC was taken as 100%.

5. Results

5.1 Interaction of donepezil with brain cystatin

Alzheimer's disease is a progressive brain disorder that gradually destroys a person's memory and ability to learn, reason, and make judgments. AChE is responsible for degradation of the neurotransmitter acetylcholine (ACh) in the synaptic cleft of neuromuscular junctions and of neuronal contacts in the central nervous system [22, 23]. Donepezil belongs to the important class of acetylcholinesterase inhibitors (AChEIs) [24]. The results of the interaction of donepezil with cystatin are given below.

5.2 Intrinsic fluorescence studies of cystatin in the presence of donepezil

Cystatin (1 μM) was incubated with various concentrations of donepezil varying from 2 to 10 μM for 30 min. The fluorescence was recorded in the wavelength region of 300–400 nm after exciting the protein solution at 280 nm for total protein fluorescence. Donepezil caused unfolding of the cystatin as indicated by enhancement in fluorescence intensity accompanied by the red shift of 40 nm as compared to –max of native cystatin (340 nm), while the drug (native) shows –max at 370 nm. However at 1.6 μM, when it forms complex with cystatin, there was a shift in –max of 10 nm with significant enhancement in fluorescence intensity (**Figure 4**).

Cystatin (1 μM) was incubated with various concentrations of donepezil varying from 0.16 to 1.6 μM for 30 min. The fluorescence was taken in the range of wavelength 300–400 nm after exciting the protein solution at 280 nm for total protein fluorescence. The slits were set at 10 nm for excitation and emission. The path length of the sample was 1 cm in the final reaction volume of 1 mL in 0.05 M sodium phosphate buffer pH 7.5.

5.3 UV-vis spectra of cystatin in the presence and absence of donepezil

Cystatin concentrations were fixed at 1 μM, while the donepezil concentrations varied from 0.16 to 1.6 μM. Absorption spectra of native cystatin and in the presence and absence of donepezil were recorded in the range of 200–300 nm. The UV absorption intensity of cystatin increased with increasing concentration of donepezil concentration; however, the slight decrease in absorption intensity may be due to disruption or perturbation of absorbing groups (**Figure 5**).

5.4 Inhibitory activity of cystatin in the presence of donepezil

A change in the inhibitory activity of cystatin with increasing concentration of donepezil is shown in **Table 1**. The effect of donepezil on cystatin function was assessed by monitoring its changes in antiproteolytic activity by caseinolytic assay of papain [21]; 1 μM of cystatin was incubated with increasing concentration of

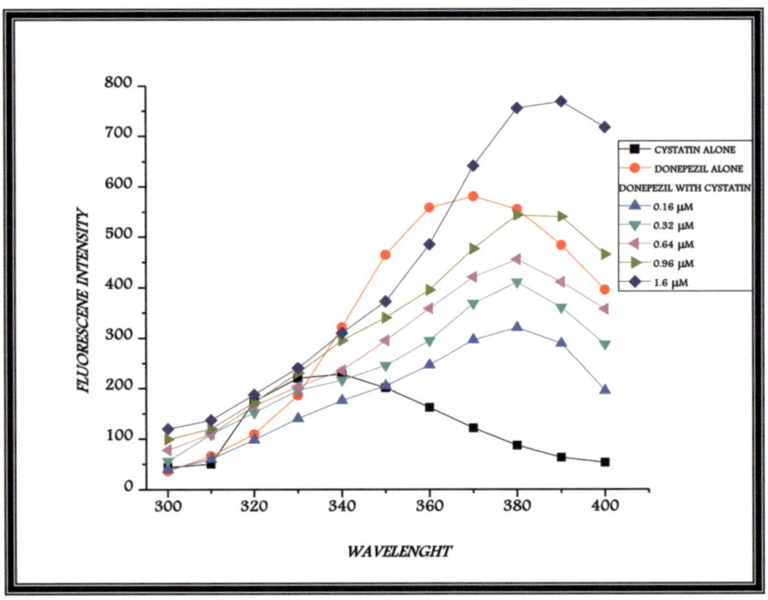

Figure 4.
Fluorescence spectra of cystatin in the presence and absence of donepezil. Cystatin (1 μM) was incubated with various concentration of Donepezil varying from 0.16 to 1.6 μM for 30 min. The fluorescence was recorded in the wavelength region 300–400 nm after exciting the protein solution at 280 nm for total protein fluorescence. The slits were set at 10 nm for excitation and emission. The path length of the sample was 1 cm in the final reaction volume of 1 ml in 0.05 M sodium phosphate buffer pH 7.5.

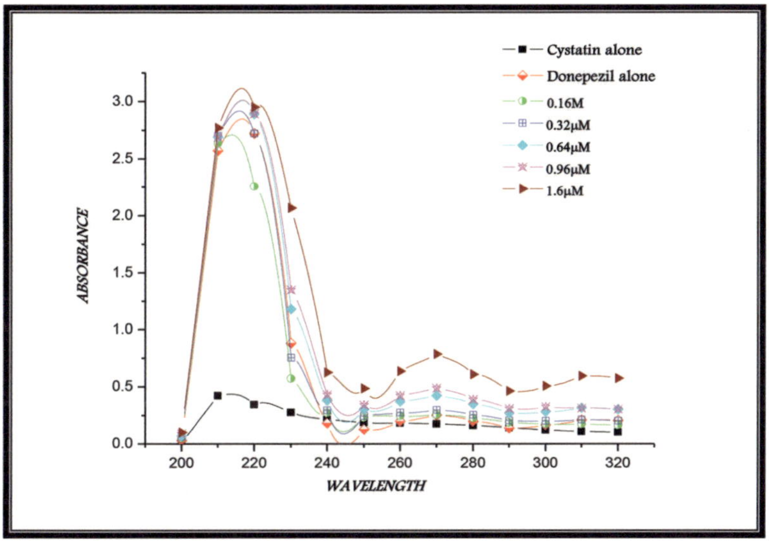

Figure 5.
UV-vis spectra of cystatin in the presence and absence of donepezil. Cystatin concentrations were fixed at 1 μM, while the donepezil concentration was varied from 0.16 to 1.6 μM. Absorption spectra of native cystatin in the presence and absence of donepezil were recorded in the range of 200–300 nm cuvette of 1 cm path length for 30 min in the final reaction volume of 1 ml in 0.05 M sodium phosphate buffer pH 7.5.

donepezil (0.16–1.6 μM). Exposure of cystatin to increasing concentration of donepezil resulted in rapid decline of antiproteolytic activity; 85% decline in the activity was seen at 1.6 μM of donepezil with more than half of the inactivation of cystatin which was taking place at concentration as low as 0.32 μM.

Table 1 shows changes in the inhibitory activity of brain cystatin after its incubation for its inhibitory activity with increasing concentrations of donepezil. Cystatin (1 μM) was treated with varying concentrations of donepezil (0.16–1.6 μM) for 30 min in the final reaction volume of 1 mL in 0.05 M sodium phosphate buffer pH 7.5.

5.5 2-D gel electrophoresis

Purity of brain cystatin was confirmed by 2-D gel electrophoresis; purified cystatin was run in one dimension on the isoelectric focusing, and after this, it was run in second dimension on 12.5% PAGE. On 2-D gel electrophoresis, BC migrated as a single

S.no	Drug concentration	% Remaining inhibitory activity of cystatin
1	Cystatin alone	100
2	Cystatin + 0.16 μM donepezil	57 ± 0.623
3	Cystatin + 0.32 μM donepezil	40 ± 0.938
4	Cystatin + 0.64 μM donepezil	38 ± 0.772
5	Cystatin + 0.96 μM donepezil	24 ± 0.932
6	Cystatin + 1.6 μM donepezil	15 ± 0.680

All data are expressed as mean ± SE for three different sets of experiments; statistical significance was conducted employing one-way ANOVA. A probability level of 0.05 was selected showing that results are significant.
The table shows changes in the inhibitory activity of brain cystatin after its incubation for its inhibitory activity with increasing concentrations of donepezil. Cystatin (1 μM) is treated with varying concentrations of donepezil (0.16–1.6 μM) for 30 min in the final reaction volume of 1 ml in 0.05 M sodium phosphate buffer pH 7.5.

Table 1.
Inhibitory activity of cystatin in the presence of donepezil.

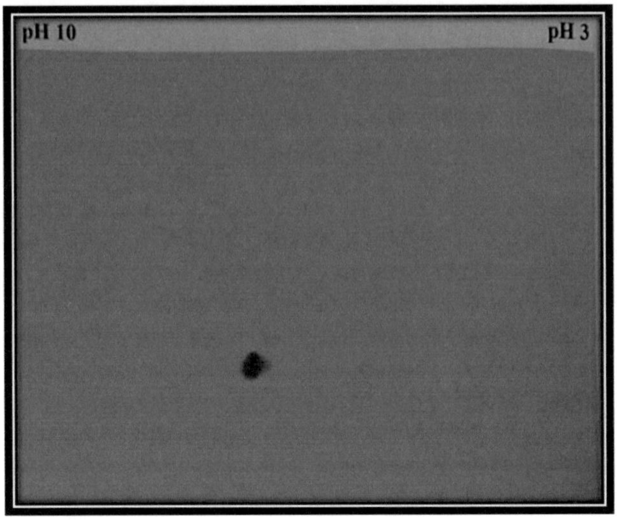

Figure 6.
2-D gel electrophoresis of purified BC: after isoelectric focusing, IPG was run horizontally over 12.5% gel between the glass slabs. A single dot was obtained toward the negative side of the IPG strip.

dot further supporting the purity nature of BC. The position of the spot was approximately in the range of 7–8 pH on IPF strip (pH 3–10) suggesting the pl of BC as 7–8.

All data are expressed as mean ± SE for three different sets of experiments; statistical significance was conducted employing one-way ANOVA. A probability level of 0.05 was selected showing that results are significant (**Figure 6**).

6. Discussion

The drug inducing changes in protein function leading to adverse side effects is the area of continual scientific investigation [25, 26].

Even small structural differences in protein conformation can lead to drastic changes in functional parameters [26]. Addition of small molecules such as many drugs, particularly those with local anesthetics, tranquilizers, and antidepressants, can bind to the native state and can alter the delicate balance of various interactions in proteins [27–30].

The adverse drug reactions are triggered due to gathering of drug molecules at localized sites in the body causing their elevated concentration [31] and ligand-induced protein structure conformational changes [32]. The drugs used as medical therapy are unable to act in the specified area because of these intricate mechanisms; therefore, all the varied external parameters are taken into account which combine the study of the conformational modifications in proteins along with drugs resulting complexes causing any side effect which are paramount for the study. These studies enable us to understand how ligand affinity can be planned and how the protein conformation upon complexation can be managed [26] which is decisive in a massive range of imperative biochemical phenomena.

In the present work and structural and functional analyses of cystatin, a protein ubiquitously present in mammalian cells and tissues was studied which showed a significant increase in fluorescence intensity due to unfolding of cystatin in the presence of donepezil (**Figure 4**). Such kind of changes have also been documented earlier, after interaction of ligands (phytohormones, cytokinins, abscisic and gibberellic acids) with wheat germ agglutinin resulting in 60% increase in fluorescence intensity of native protein [33].

Donepezil-cystatin complexation showed 40 nm red shift in λ_{max} indicating exposure of aromatic residues to the solvent caused by conformational changes in the protein [34, 35]. Absorption spectral measurements of cystatin in the presence of drug showed a peak noticeable at 275 and 210 nm in spectra obtained at 0.16 μM donepezil concentration (**Figure 5**). Suggesting changes mainly due to tryptophan and tyrosine residues [36].

Thus, the results indicate that the UV absorption and fluorescence emission changes in donepezil-mediated interaction are due to conformational changes in cystatin mainly arising from interaction affecting the chromophoric groups of the protein which produce significant effect on the activity of cystatin. The study shows that in the presence of donepezil, cystatin gets unfolded which is a side effect of donepezil.

There is a gradual decline in the cystatin activity with increasing drug concentration resulting in 62% loss at 0.64 μM donepezil (**Table 1**). Further magnitude of decline was relatively smaller with increasing drug concentration up to 1.6 μM. Cystatin retained only 15% of its antiproteolytic potential.

The knowledge about the pharmacokinetics and pharmacodynamics of the drug-protein interaction continues to expand. The increased information available to clinicians might help in optimizing the use of these agents in the management of patients with Alzheimer's disease and other diseases. The clinical utility of measuring these parameters in daily practice awaits further research [37].

Author details

Fakhra Amin[1] and Bilqees Bano[2]*

1 Department of Zoology, Faculty of Life Sciences, Aligarh Muslim University, Aligarh, Uttar Pradesh, India

2 Department of Biochemistry, Faculty of Life Sciences, Aligarh Muslim University, Aligarh, Uttar Pradesh, India

*Address all correspondence to: bilqeesbano691@gmail.com

References

[1] Bernstein HG, Kirschke H, Wiederanders B, Pollak KH, Zipress A, Rinne A. The possible place of cathepsins and cystatins in the puzzle of Alzheimer disease. Molecular and Chemical Neuropathology. 1996;**27**(3):225-247. Review. PubMed PMID: 9147410.10

[2] Birks JS, Melzer D, Beppu H. Donepezil for mild and moderate Alzheimer's disease. Cochrane Database of Systematic Reviews. 2000;**4**:CD001190. Review. PubMed PMID: 11034704

[3] Sugimoto H, OguraH AY, Limura Y, Yamanishi Y. Research and development of donepezil hydrochloride, a new type of acetylcholinesterase inhibitor. The Japanese Journal of Pharmacology. 2002;**89**(1):7-20. Review. PubMed PMID: 12083745

[4] German DC, Yazdani U, Speciale SG, Pasbakhsh P, Games D, Liang CL. Cholinergic neuropathology in a mouse model of Alzheimer's disease. The Journal of Comparative Neurology. 2003;**462**(4):371-381. PubMed PMID: 12811807

[5] Yamanishi Y, Ogura H, Kosasa T, Araki S, Sawa Y, Yamatsu K. Inhibitory action of E2020, a novel acetylcholinesterase inhibitor, on cholinesterase: Comparison with other inhibitors. In: Nagatsu T, editor. Basic, Clinical, and Therapeutic Aspects of Alzheimer's and Parkinson's Diseases. Vol. 2. New York: Plenum Press; 1991. pp. 409-413

[6] Sugimoto H, Iimura Y, Yamanishi Y, Yamatsu K. Synthesis and structure-activity relationships of acetylcholinesterase inhibitors: 1-benzyl-4-[(5,6-dimethoxy-1-oxoindan-2-yl)methyl]piperidine hydrochloride and related compounds. Journal of Medicinal Chemistry. 1995;**38**:4821-4829

[7] Mihara M, Ohnishi A, Tomono Y, Hasegawa J, Shimamura Y, Yamazaki K, et al. Pharmacokinetics of E2020, a new compound for Alzheimer's disease, in healthy male volunteers. International Journal of Clinical Pharmacology and Therapeutics. 1993;**31**:223-229

[8] Rogers SL, Farlow MR, Doody RS, Mohs R, Friedhoff L. T and the donepezil study group. A 24-week, double-blind, placebo-controlled trial of donepezil in patients with Alzheimer's disease. Neurology. 1998;**50**:136-145

[9] Rogers SL, Doody RS, Mohs R, Friedhoff L. T and the donepezil study group. Donepezil improves cognitive and global function in Alzheimer's disease: A 15-week double-blind, placebo controlled study. Archives of Internal Medicine. 1998;**158**:1021-1031

[10] Birks J, Harvey RJ. Donepezil for dementia due to Alzheimer's disease. Cochrane Database of Systematic Reviews. 2006;**25**(1):CD001190. Review. PubMed PMID: 16437430

[11] Jann MW, Shirley KL, Small GW. Clinical pharmacokinetics and pharmacodynamics of cholinesterase inhibitors. Clinical Pharmacokinetics. 2002;**41**(10):719-739. Review. PubMed PMID: 12162759

[12] Bernstein HG, Wiederanders B. An immunohistochemical study of cathepsin E in Alzheimer-type dementia brains. Brain Research. 1994;**667**(2):287-290. PubMed PMID: 7697369

[13] Ekiel I, Abrahamson M, Fulton DB, Lindahl P, Storer AC, Levadoux W, et al. NMR structural studies of human cystatin C dimers and monomers. Journal of Molecular Biology. 1997;**271**(2):266-277. PubMed PMID: 9268658

[14] Cox JL. Cystatins and cancer. Frontiers in Bioscience. 2009;**14**:463-474. Review. PubMed PMID: 19273078

[15] Grzonka Z, Jankowska E, Kasprzykowski F, Kasprzykowska R, Lankiewicz L, Wiczk W, et al. Structural studies of cysteine proteases and their inhibitors. Acta Biochimica Polonica. 2001;**48**(1):1-20. Review. PubMed PMID: 11440158

[16] Levy E. Cystatin C: A potential target for Alzheimer's treatment. Expert Review of Neurotherapeutics. 2008;**8**(5):687-689. Review. PubMed PMID: 18457524

[17] Gotti R, Bertucci C, Andrisano V, Pomponio R, Cavrini V. Study of donepezil binding to serum albumin by capillary electrophoresis and circular dichroism. Analytical and Bioanalytical Chemistry. 2003;**377**(5):875-879. PubMed PMID: 12955395

[18] Turk V, Turk B. Lysosomal cysteine proteases and their protein inhibitors: Recent developments. Acta Chimica Slovenica—A Review. 2008;**55**:727-738

[19] Shah A, Bano B. Cystatins in health and diseases. International Journal of Peptide Research and Therapeutics. 2008;**15**:43-48. DOI: 10.1007/s10989-008-9160-1

[20] Amin F, Khan AA, Rizvi SJ, Bano B. Purification and characterization of buffalo brain cystatin. Protein and Peptide Letters. 2011;**18**(2):210-218. PubMed PMID: 21054269

[21] Kunitz M. Crystalline soybean trypsin inhibitor II. General properties. The Journal of General Physiology. 1947;**30**:291-310

[22] Kasa P, Papp H, Kasa P Jr, Torok I. Donepezil dose-dependently inhibits acetylcholinesterase activity in various areas and in the presynaptic cholinergic and the postsynaptic cholinoceptive enzyme-positive structures in the human and rat brain. Neuroscience. 2000;**101**(1):89-100. PubMed PMID: 11068139

[23] Tabet N. Acetylcholinesterase inhibitors for Alzheimer's disease: Anti-inflammatories in acetylcholine clothing! Age and Ageing. 2006;**35**(4):336-338. PubMed PMID: 16788077

[24] Kaur J, Zhang MQ. Molecular modelling and QSAR of reversible acetylcholinesterase inhibitors. Current Medicinal Chemistry. 2000;**7**(3):273-294. Review. PubMed PMID: 10637365

[25] Priyamvada S, Priyadarshini M, Arivarasu NA, Farooq N, Khan S, Khan SA, et al. Studies on the protective effect of dietary fish oil on gentamicin-induced nephrotoxicity and oxidative damage in rat kidney. Prostaglandins, Leukotrienes, and Essential Fatty Acids. 2008;**78**(6):369-381. PubMed PMID: 18556188

[26] Sneppen K, Zocchi G. Physics in Molecular Biology. 1st ed. Cambridge University Press; 2005. ISBN: 0-521-84419-3

[27] Salvi A, Carrupt P, Tillement J, Testa B. Structural damage to proteins caused by free radicals: Assessment, protection by antioxidants, and influence of protein binding. Biochemical Pharmacology. 2001;**61**(10):1237-1242. PubMed PMID: 11322927

[28] Guo M, Zou JW, Yi PG, Shang ZC, Hu GX, Yu QS. Binding interaction of gatifloxacin with bovine serum albumin. Analytical Sciences. 2004;**20**(3):465-470. PubMed PMID: 15068289

[29] Cheema MA, Taboada P, Barbosa S, Gutiérrez-Pichel M, Castro E, Siddiq M, et al. Energetics of binding and protein unfolding upon amphiphilic

drug complexation with a globular protein in different aqueous media. Colloids and Surfaces. B, Biointerfaces. 2008;**63**(2):217-228. PubMed PMID: 18222070

[30] Ahmed-Ouameur A, Diamantoglou S, Sedaghat-Herati MR, Nafisi S, Carpentier R, Tajmir-Riahi HA. The effects of drug complexation on the stability and conformation of human serum albumin: Protein unfolding. Cell Biochemistry and Biophysics. 2006;**45**(2):203-213. Review. PubMed PMID: 16757821

[31] Wen ZM, Ye ST. Skin testing in patients with high risk of anaphylactic reactions to penicillin. Asian Pacific Journal of Allergy and Immunology. 1993;**11**(1):13-18. PubMed PMID: 8216554

[32] Takeda K, Wada A, Yamamoto K, Hachiya K, Batra Prem P. Secondary structure change of myoglobin induced by sodium dodecyl sulfate and its kinetic aspects. Journal of Colloid and Interface Science. 1988;**125**(1):307-313. Available online 21 July 2004

[33] Bogoeva VP, Radeva MA, Atanasova LY, Stoitsova SR, Boteva RN. Fluorescence analysis of hormone binding activities of wheat germ agglutinin. Biochimica et Biophysica Acta. 2004;**1698**(2):213-218. PubMed PMID: 15134654

[34] Monsellier E, Bedouelle H. Quantitative measurement of protein stability from unfolding equilibria monitored with the fluorescence maximum wavelength. Protein Engineering, Design & Selection. 2005;**18**(9):445-456. PubMed PMID: 16087653

[35] Vivian JT, Callis PR. Mechanisms of tryptophan fluorescence shifts in proteins. Biophysical Journal. 2001;**80**(5):2093-2109. PubMed PMID: 11325713

[36] Donovan JW. Ultraviolet difference spectroscopy–New techniques and applications. Methods in Enzymology. 1973;**27**:497-525. PubMed PMID: 4773294

[37] Crismon ML. Pharmacokinetics and drug interactions of cholinesterase inhibitors administered in Alzheimer's disease. Pharmacotherapy. 1998; **47-54**:79-82. Review. PubMed PMID: 9543465

Section 3

Pharmaceutical Limits in Therapeutic Options

Chapter 5

Non-pharmacological Treatment of Alzheimer's

Terezia Fertalova and Iveta Ondriova

Abstract

Caring for a patient with dementia is challenging, as we cannot cure Alzheimer's disease but only slow its progress. In the presented chapter, we offer non-pharmacological approaches for influencing the patient's behaviour, actions and emotions, and to arouse their interest and motivation, while preserving the highest quality of life. In the past, many experts have looked at specific approaches to dementia patients and devoted their entire professional lives to senior citizens. Our aim is to offer an overview of the most frequently used therapeutic approaches with dementia patients and use practical demonstrations to reinvigorate the theoretical basis. At the end of the chapter we deal with the burden on the carer in the family environment.

Keywords: Alzheimer's disease, memory, non-pharmacological, treatment, carer

1. Introduction

With the increasing number of seniors, the number of newly diagnosed patients with dementia syndrome, including Alzheimer's disease, is rising. At the same time, the costs of treatment are increasing. This has led experts to focus on less costly, non-pharmacological treatment of dementia.

Examining non-pharmacological approaches to patients with dementia and their family carers does not have such a long tradition or history as the scientific examination of pharmacological approaches. Certainly, scientists have always taken it as given that besides pharmacotherapy, it is useful to activate, reassure, adapt the environment and other procedures experienced by non-medical staff in particular. These procedures have long been considered appropriate and useful, but not too stimulating or interesting for further scientific research. However, in the last decade, work has appeared examining non-pharmacological approaches to dementia patients and their family members [1].

The goal of non-pharmacological treatment is to maintain or improve the level of gross and fine motor skills, walking, self-sufficiency and cognitive functions. At the same time, another goal is to meaningfully fill free time and to influence the symptoms of dementia and activities of daily life, to improve verbal and non-verbal communication between the sufferer and their relative or nurse....

The activities we choose must be appropriate to the condition of the sufferer. There are multiple non-pharmacological approaches; the therapist selects from a spectrum of options, taking into account the age of the patient, the stage of the disease, the gender, therefore it is necessary to emphasize the individual approach.

Activities should be comprehensive, adequately influence the mental and physical aspects and the psychosocial contacts. Activities should always promote the patient's strengths. It is important to have a familiar environment for the patient. The process of the activities themselves is important. An activity that does not come off successfully does not mean a loss. Treatment of this type should become a regular part of the daily regimen of a patient with dementia [2].

Non-pharmacological approaches to dementia management focus on the following problem areas:

- Early diagnosis and patient support in the initial phase of the disease.
- Providing information, preserving or improving cognitive functions.
- Preservation or improvement of the patient's self-sufficiency.
- Mitigating or eliminating problematic behaviour and the psychological symptoms of dementia.
- Improving the quality of life for the patient with dementia.
- Improving the communication between the patient and the doctor treating them.
- Improving the quality of life of patients in the terminal stages of dementia.
- Support for carers [3].

The aim of our work is to summarize current theoretical knowledge about non-pharmacological approaches with patients with Alzheimer's disease and to illustrate examples of the implementation of specific approaches. When formulating the theoretical basis, we used the available specialist and scientific publications. The practical examples are the result of qualitative research aimed at verifying activation approaches for Alzheimer's disease patients.

Caring for a patient with Alzheimer's disease requires that we recognize the basic principles and recommendations for care.

2. Non-pharmacological treatment of Alzheimer's

A regular daytime routine is an important part of care for a patient with dementia because in the advanced stages of dementia, patients benefit from a certain regularity of the daily routine. A natural rhythm comes from the time of eating, time for leisure activities or for hygiene. If we offer a variety of options to the patient and we program the individual activities for specific days, we fill the patient's time meaningfully, thereby preventing periods of troubles. Overly interesting or too many activities can have the opposite effect, so we emphasize the individual approach and accepting the patient's abilities.

Nutritional support is part of comprehensive therapy and has an important place in the comprehensive treatment of dementia patients. Nutritional care can improve the results of treatment [4]. Epidemiological and clinical studies abroad have shown that dietary supplements can reduce the risk of cognitive impairment and greatly improve its further course. Aging individuals who consume enough fish (sea fish two to three times a week) and fish products, omega-3 fatty acids and *Ginkgo biloba* see an effect on their cognitive function which can slow down the development of cognitive deficits [5]. Walnuts are an important part of nutrition for a patient with dementia. They are rich in protein, vitamins, omega 3 fatty acids, trace elements, lecithin and oils. Walnuts are an important part of the diet with regard to brain activity. Compared to other nuts, which usually contain a large amount of monounsaturated fatty acids, walnuts contain especially polyunsaturated fatty acids. They have only a negligible amount of sodium and are free of cholesterol. They also contain enough folic acid and thiamine and a useful amount of vitamin E in the form of tocopherol. They contain manganese, magnesium, phosphorus and iron. The folk saying is that walnuts have the shape of a brain so they undoubtedly support the health of the brain [6, 7].

Apples, spinach, extra virgin olive oil, grape juice and red wine, salmon, curry pepper and curcumin, cinnamon, coffee and hot chocolate improve brain activity and have a preventive effect.

When stretching our thinking or memory, we lean towards the substances that irritate the nervous system. They are sometimes called 'memory poisons'. These substances stimulate the current intellectual capacity and improve memory and focus. Substances like this include: caffeine, nicotine, alcohol, calming drugs (tranquilizers) [8].

Leading the patient towards self-sufficiency is an important principle in the care of a dementia patient. All care providers should be sufficiently qualified and have the patience to use gradual steps, instruction and help to lead patients to perform their own care by themselves. This approach too must be applied sensitively, with knowledge of the condition and the patient's capabilities, the patient cannot be expected to perform activities that they are no longer able to do. This approach is recommended in the mild and moderate stages of the disease.

Patient activation is understood the preservation and improvement of their capabilities by assigning different tasks. Particularly, pet therapy is more of a home-based type of therapy when the dementia patient's level of activity is maintained by looking after a pet [9].

Orientation in reality is one of the oldest approaches to patients. At present, only some elements of orientation in reality are used. This approach, if applied consistently and thoroughly, improves patient orientation but at the cost of total discomfort [10]. Nowadays, orientation in reality is used mainly in the initial stages of Alzheimer's disease when the patient has short-term losses of memory. The patient has a calendar, saying the day, month, year, their name, address, and other information that would return them to reality during a short-term loss of memory. Suitable approaches include the colour coding of rooms and the use of pictograms to improve the spatial orientation of the patient. Orientation in reality is important in the light and moderate stages of the illness, when the patient experiences memory loss, and aids can be used to orient them in the real situation.

Programming activities is suitable for people undergoing advanced dementia. The progression of the disease leads to a worsening of the overall condition, when patients need the most individualized care. In the event that the individual activities burden the patient, we stop trying to force their active participation and adapt to the specific pace, needs and possibilities of the patient. Programming activities is an important part of care in the advanced stage of the disease and it can be said that it is to a great extent a specific need at this stage of the disease [10].

Milieu therapy is also known as environmental manipulation. Its use is appropriate in the mild and moderate stage of Alzheimer's disease. It is a comprehensive individual approach to the patient and the adaptation of the environment in which they function so that they feel pleasant and can better orient themselves through plenty of sensory stimuli provided. Some facilities for seniors that are specially designed for dementia patients accept this concept in advance. In particular, it is important for the patient to be easily orientated in the interior. One problem may be, for example, an unusual design for flushing the toilet, which the patient may not know or the taps/faucets. Sometimes it is advisable to camouflage the entrance door, for example with wallpaper, so as not to tempt the patient to leave the ward. The space should be stable and should change as little as possible [10].

Practical demonstration:

In the gerontological psychiatry ward, patients' rooms were numbered. Patients found it harder to orient themselves in this space and often did not return to their room. When the door of the room was marked with pictures of fruit (pear, apple, plum, banana, oranges), it turned out that the orientation of the patient in the space was easier.

Lifestyle approach is sharing information among care providers. Patients may have different individual habits, which should also be accepted during dementia. They include the daily routine of the patient, their habits, way of dressing, using the toilet, the activities they perform by themselves, and those for which they need help. If the treating staff respect long-followed habits and rituals, it will facilitate care. Failure to do this often causes aggression, unrest, and other situations that lead to a worsening of the patient's condition. Some facilities have questionnaires, entry interviews to this end, which aim to get as much detail as possible. If the attending staff does not accept routine habits and rituals, it usually increases the aggressive behaviour of the patient. Practice shows that the experience of family carers is a valuable aid in the care of the sick [10].

Practical demonstration:

In a social care facility for the elderly, a patient did not evacuate into the toilet but always onto the floor. Repeated instructions from the treating staff did not help, nor did labelling the toilet with a pictogram. Unpleasant and bewildering situations occurred like this. In a deeper study into why the patient does not accept evacuating into the toilet, it was found that the patient was from a socially deprived environment and he only began using a toilet during adulthood. By simple intervention—removing the toilet door and the coloured curtain at the entrance to the toilet, the patient was able to learn where to evacuate. Another solution to the situation could be, for example, the use of a disposable diaper, which would be uncomfortable for the patient, but would facilitate the work of the attending staff. An individual approach can also bring about an easy solution to a seemingly simple situation.

2.1 Cognitive training

In the following section we list non-pharmacological approaches to dementia patients. For each approach, we provide practical examples of how we have used them in the care of patients with dementia.

Cognitive training is targeted stimulation of brain functions with a focus on multiple cognitive abilities. It is mainly used in initial and middle stage Alzheimer's patients who want to train their cognitive skills by themselves. It slows the development of the disease and improves the quality of life. Sometimes it also serves as a daily activity or fun, depending on how the patient takes it. Studies have shown that in some patients in the moderate and serious stages of the disease cognitive training leads to negative reactions, such as depression and frustration [11]. We can use the techniques of cognitive training in ordinary life. For example, we can go shopping without a shopping list, solve mathematical problems without a calculator, sometimes we can even learn something 'by heart' such as a song or poem, or we can imitate the main actors after a film has ended [12]. Cognitive training has a particularly important role to play in preventing cognitive decline, strengthening self-esteem, self-confidence, promoting self-sufficiency in day-to-day activities, helping maintain quality of life, promoting social contacts, and enhancing welfare and enjoyment of success [13]. The worst thing for memory is inactivity and a lack of stimuli for processing. If the memory is not regularly stimulated it gets 'lazy' and its functioning worsens, just like another organ or muscle [12].

Practical demonstration:

Example 1: An 81-year-old patient has observed over several years that her memory is getting worse and she forgets everything quickly. She forgets everything she wants to buy or take out of the refrigerator, she does not remember her relatives' birthdays and other special days. All her information and appointments must be written in a calendar or diary. She does smaller shopping trips on her own, but she always has to prepare a shopping ticket. The client leads an active life. Every day she goes for 30-minute walks, which promotes brain oxygenation and supports memory functions. She attends university of the third-age and a retirees' club, where she gets new enthusiasm and meets people. She reads books every day, does crosswords, watches quizzes on television. These day-to-day activities are a natural part of the daily life of an active senior which stimulate cognitive functions and train the brain in an unforced way.

Example 2: In a retirement home, seniors trained their memory functions. As an activity they chose preparing food. Patients under the supervision of their therapist, remembered a variety of different recipes, specifically for: pancakes. Because they are in a social care facility and are not preparing meals themselves they had to think more deeply about recipes. Together, they agreed on a recipe which they then prepared under the supervision of the therapist.

This activation is an example of how we could implement cognitive training without realizing it and it can become a natural part of the daily program of senior citizens in institutionalized care.

2.2 Snoezelen therapy

Snoezelen therapy is a multifunctional method that is performed in a particularly pleasant and adapted environment. This therapy offers patients with dementia a suitable alternative solution with the ability to become aware of their surroundings. It allows them to better respond to the environment they are part of. The stimulating environment helps to reduce aggression and improve the mood just by calming the body and mind, so it can induce inner balance and peace. Through stimuli, such as sound and light effects, relaxing music, tactile surfaces, or the pleasant smell of essential oil, it stimulates external senses such as hearing, sight, touch, smell or taste. It creates an environment that creates nice and pleasant memories, and it also helps stimulate and activate old habits [14].

Snoezelen is the name for a multi-sensory room that provides beautiful sensory experiences using technology that generates sensual responses and reactions from the client. This room produces a sense of well-being, it releases and relaxes, activates and awakes the senses. But it also provokes memories, directs and unites stimuli, destroys fear, brings security, reduces aggression, self-destruction and violent behaviour [15].

When using Snoezelen therapy, it is not possible to determine in advance how the patient will respond. Even if it makes us feel comfortable, we can equally expect the opposite reaction. Multi-sensory stimulation is recommended at least once or twice a week with an interval of at least 30 minutes to prevent the patient from becoming saturated with stimuli. Snoezelen therapy is appropriate in all stages of dementia, but it is especially beneficial if we are interested in a patient in a severe stage and we can stimulate the psyche and arouse pleasant feelings.

Practical demonstration of a negative reaction:

An 86-year-old patient with a severe degree of Alzheimer's dementia does not recognize his relatives, he is limited in movement, speaks incomprehensibly, sleeps during the day and is restless at night. At the entrance to the Snoezelen room, the patient sharpened his gaze and began to look around. The patient was placed in the centre of the room in the wheelchair, we began the light effects: bubble cylinders, starry sky, we quietly turned on the music. Through his knees, we passed interactive optical fibers that he touched with his hands. The patient was silent for about 10 minutes, observing the surroundings, playing with the interactive fibers in his hands. After a while the patient began to be nervous, he was fidgeting, he lowered his eyes, and muttered something quietly. After a while, he started to shout nonsensically. He was aggressive. We finished the Snoezelen therapy.

In repeat therapies, the patient responded in the same manner, so we will not use this multisensory stimulus for the specific patient, but we will choose another non-pharmacological approach.

2.3 Reminiscence therapy

Reminiscence therapy is a method that uses memories and their recall using various stimuli. Of course, it is also suitable for healthy seniors, for its preventive and activating significance. It is mainly useful for patients with dementia, who have short-term memory disorders, but conversely, they are often have surprisingly good recall of events from the past [3].

Reminiscence therapy typically refers to a therapist's conversation with an elderly person (or group) about their life up to that point, their past activities, events and experiences, often using appropriate tools (old photographs, objects, tools and home appliances, and old working tools, fashion accessories, movies, folk or dance music, and so on). The activity may be more or less structured, but also completely spontaneous, unstructured, with the therapeutic aspect sometimes coming more or less to the fore. The use of reminiscence is especially useful for people with dementia, when it comes to reviving past experiences, especially those that are positively and personally important, such as family events, holidays, weddings, celebrations, etc. [16].

This type of therapy uses memories and stimulates their recall using various stimuli. Its goal is to improve the overall state and strengthen human dignity, and improve communication. It can be individual or group and its methods vary, such as: viewing photo albums, watching old films, telling old stories, and other activities such as singing, reciting, etc. [17].

In some facilities, memory rooms are also available for clients, in which the interior furnishings and environmental adaptations correspond to the period of the youth of clients [18].

Practical recommendations:

In reminiscence therapy, different situations can arise that cause both positive and negative emotions, such as memories of parents, siblings, time that can no longer be returned. If the patient expresses anger or sadness, we do not have to worry about these emotions and avoid them at all costs. An individual approach is very important, because in some people the emotional expression will cause relief, while conversely in some people it will deepen their depressive mood. Aging is a natural cycle of life that must be accepted and accepted with respect and sometimes it is necessary to lead the patient to that.

If reminiscence leads to very unpleasant and painful memories, it is more appropriate to avoid such an approach.

2.4 Validation therapy

Validation therapy is considered to be one of the first specific non-pharmacological approaches to patients affected by dementia.

Considering the specifications of the procedure we devote greater attention to the theoretical basis, which should be of more benefit to the reader. The validation method was developed by Naomi Feil. Naomi Feil was born in Munich in 1932 and grew up in a retirement home where her father was the director. She was also employed by her mother, who worked there as head of the social department. After completing her studies of social work, she was awarded a Master's degree in social work, after which she started working with the elderly. Based on her dissatisfaction with the approaches and methods of old-age care of time, she began to develop a different manner of therapy. The whole development of this therapy took place between 1963 and 1980. In addition to the theoretical foundations, she developed her model primarily from her own experience. As long as she had spent almost all her life among old people, she had a lot of experience. As a child grew up among the seniors, she worked with them for 7 years. Later she worked for over 40 years with very old and confused people aged over 80.

Nowadays, the Naomi Feil Validation Concept is recognized as a method based on the latest knowledge in the care of elderly people with Alzheimer's disease, dementia or related diseases. This method is accepted in both palliative medicine and gerontology [19]. Validation is a form of communication and therapy used with old people suffering from dementia syndrome or other disorders whose manifestation is mental disorientation. It is based on the different principles of psychology, therapeutic approaches and biography [13]. The validation method is considered to be high moral support and a form of assistance we can provide to a senior with dementia syndrome. However, the springboard to providing it must be the willingness of workers to take a completely different view of this issue, to try to understand the right cause of the behaviour of disoriented seniors, and also effort and consistency in using new approaches to the patient.

Validation as such is a sensitive generalization by experts dealing with people with dementia. Its main principle is respect for the person. We do not violently oppose the misconceptions of a person with dementia, nor do we support them in that. Validating someone means accepting their emotions, telling him that their emotions are true. The refusal of emotion causes uncertainty.

The purpose of validation is to help elderly people stay as long as possible in their home environment, to restore self-confidence, to reduce stress, to make sense of life as experienced, to deal with unaddressed conflicts of the past, to improve verbal and non-verbal communication, to prevent a return to vegetation, to improve the ability to walk and physical health in general, to provide the carer with joy and energy, to help families communicate with their disoriented relatives [20].

There are several principles that a user of validation must consider if they want to perform validation therapy on old, disoriented people. One must realize a few facts:

1. Even porly oriented or disoriented seniors are unique and have their value.

2. Do not try to change them at all costs, accept them as they are.

3. We must be able to listen; empathic listening creates an environment conducive to confiding, reduces their anxiety and, above all, brings dignity.

4. Expressed, accepted and validated painful feelings become weaker. But if ignored and suppressed they remain strong.

5. There are reasons for the behaviour the poorly oriented and disoriented old people.

6. The behaviour of these people can be rooted in one or more human needs. Processing unresolved task for a peaceful and balanced death, the need to live

in peace, the need to regain their balance, as mobility memory and senses are lost, the need to give meaning to a gloomy reality, to find a place where they can feel happy, the need for status, recognition, self-sufficiency, the need to be productive and useful, the need to be respected and to belong, the need to express their feelings and be heard, the need for human contact, the need for certainty and security, not limitation, the need for any stimulation, and finally the need to reduce pain and complications.

7. In the case of failure of verbal expression and short-term memory, old learned patterns of behaviour return.

8. Things, persons, or objects of the past are replaced by personal symbols that represent them and have an emotional charge.

9. Disoriented or partially oriented seniors live at different levels of consciousness, often at the same time.

10. By weakening the five senses, these seniors can stimulate and use their own 'inner meaning', seeing through their inner vision and hearing the tones from the past.

11. Various emotions, colours, sounds, coincidences, smells, tastes and images can now awaken emotions that recall similar emotion from the past [21].

During validation, we do not quarrel with the old person and do not confront them with the opposite view, we do not try to provide a view of their behaviour, and we do not try to improve their orientation in time unless it is of interest to the old person. Individual or group therapy does not establish firm rules to target it over time. The user of validation is not perceived as an authority but as a diligent assistant.

2.4.1 Forms of validation therapy

The basic forms of validation therapy include individual and group forms. In the **individual form**, the therapist works in three steps.

1. In the first step, they collect all available information that is needed for the validation itself, but also for evaluating its effectiveness. The therapist gets information on things 'here and now' and about 'things then and there'.

2. The second step involves determining the phase in which the person is. In this step, they compare the information obtained with the individual's statements and determines the stage or phase in which the old person is located.

3. The third step is the validation therapy itself. A therapist should come regularly and use validation techniques that can help them at different stages.

Group therapy is conditional on the creation of mutual trust so that individual members can express their own feelings, communicate verbally and non-verbally, solve problems, be active in selected social roles, learn the highest possible degree of control and, in particular, to gain a feeling of their own about their own value. The goal of group validation is to reduce fear, reduce the need for limiting and calming methods, and prevent vegetation in old dementia patients. Another less important goal for relatives and staff is for validation to reduce their risk of burnout syndrome [21].

It is possible, for the best use of the validation team, to involve all workers—not only nursing staff, but also staff from cleaning, kitchens, offices, social workers or physiotherapists. The most appropriate solution is to create a validation team that would stimulate the client or patient with the same validation techniques [22].

The therapy itself in the group consists of seven steps.

The first step is getting to know the person. At this point it is necessary also to evaluate the phase or stage of disorientation in individual validation too. For the correct evaluation, it is possible to use the questionnaire 'Selecting members of the validation group' or the 'Life story and basic behaviour' form can be used. All this is necessary, because the knowing the group members is also the basis for its success.

The second step is selecting the group members. As the group is diverse, it is necessary to assemble it so that everyone has its place in it. A former clergyman can begin by praying, a former teacher of singing can lead singing. Naomi Feil exactly describes what the composition of the members should be like and at what stage of disorientation they should be. There should be five to ten people in the group—one leader personality, one wise and hospitable person, four or five people who like discussion, about two people in the third stage who could respond to the validation therapist, and two people still do not feel threatened by disoriented persons.

The third step is to find a role for each member. At each meeting an individual should play the same role, because it represents a certainty for him and promotes dignity. As an example, Naomi Feil gives an introducer, who opens and ends the meeting, a singer who sets the rhythm and conducts, someone who reads in the group, the person who prepares the chairs, the flowers, the secretary, the host.

In **the fourth step**, it is appropriate to involve all the staff in the validation. This can help with preparation and implementation. They can provide a room and/or refreshment, bring individual members of the group, and suggest new members or new topics.

The fifth step is music itself, the discussion, movement, eating. The music should start and end the session, and one song is enough. For the discussion, it is advisable to choose the topics in advance—the loss of a loved one, home or work, boredom, searching for a new sense of life.

The sixth step is to schedule a meeting. This step consists not only of a meeting plan, but also of the preparation of materials and room, of the timetable and all the information available to help the meeting.

In **the seventh step** is meeting itself alone. It should be done at least once a week at the same time and in the same place. It is composed of four parts—introduction, life, conclusion and preparation of the next meeting [21]. The basis for validation meetings is how and what a person with dementia really wants to express themselves, and even if it does not coincide with reality, appropriately and adequately respond to it [23].

Practical demonstration:

An 82-year-old patient in a severe stage of Alzheimer's disease was admitted to the psychiatric ward. The patient was disoriented in time and space. The patient had an increased risk of falls due to his advanced age and limited mobility. The patient used antipsychotics and sedatives. Hospitalization was necessary because in the domestic environment the patient was always going away, not accepting the guidance of the carers, he was restless at night, he shouted. During hospitalization, despite the psychopharmaceuticals, the patient's behaviour did not change. During the day he was restless, always wanting to go home, he ran out of the room. The treating staff constantly focused on reality and reminded him that he was hospitalized, could not go home, must lie in bed...The patient's behaviour was difficult to handle. According to the Naomi Feil validation concept, we are not trying to improve his orientation, we do not argue and do not confront him with the opposite view. We tried to use these recommendations in communicating with the patient. If the patient requested to go home, we did not give him the reasons why he could not go home and where he was, but we turned the communication in a different direction. We asked why he wanted to go home, what he would do at home, what he used to do outside in the garden, with whom he met...The patient began to talk about what he used to do at home and where he worked. This does not mean that the patient was getting better, but he lightened his tone in communication, he did not shout, after a group walk around the department, the patient could be directed and was sitting quietly in the chair.

We have found a way how we can influence patient behaviour and actions....

2.5 Doll therapy

Doll therapy is a very effective form of comprehensive therapy in patients with various forms and degrees of dementia, mental retardation, physical disability, and various psychiatric disorders. It is known for its low financial burden and easy accessibility. The therapeutic dolls resemble young children in terms of their size and appearance. Dolls are made with natural material, which is also anti-allergic. To touch it is pleasant, soft and positively stimulates the patient's senses. The individual body parts are specially balanced for better handling. The legs are malleable, suitable for enveloping the patient and encouraging hugging. Such manipulation is used as part of basal stimulation. The indirect gaze of all the dolls (eyes do not look ahead) is deliberately neutral. It feels peaceful to the patients and does not cause negative emotions. Doll therapy is based on long-term memory paths. It is normal that these patients, especially women, are looking for their children and want to take care of something or someone. It is through dolls that we try to stimulate this ability. Furthermore, we try to stimulate fine motor skills, nerve activity, especially attention, memory, supporting patient activity, dialog, establishing relationships, inducing a sense of security, love and peace. In some cases, the use of psychopharmaceuticals has been reduced.

The use of dolls with a patient is associated with a number of benefits that include increasing welfare, inducing positive emotions, good sleep, improving eating habits, reducing agitation, irritability, anxiety episodes, apathy, depression, aggression and tension by distraction towards a substitute, improving communication and sociability. In spite of the benefits, the use of therapeutic dolls also has its negatives, such as the infantilization of the senior, thereby breaking ethics. For these reasons, we must emphasize the individual approach and we cannot generalize their mass use under any circumstances [24].

Before starting to use therapeutic dolls with a patient with Alzheimer's disease, it is necessary to train the attending staff or relatives. It is essential to realize the benefits and potential problems that may arise over time. Success also depends on the attitude of the staff. In the case of an uncommitted or negative attitude on the part of the staff, success will usually not occur. Before starting doll therapy, one needs to get some fundamental information about their role as a mother or father, because sometimes negative experiences in the life of the patient may render the use of doll therapy inappropriate. This is, for example, the death of a child, a severely ill child, or a child not interested in the parent....

Each patient should have their own doll. It is recommended to find out whether the patient had a son or daughter, to find their hair colour and choose the type of doll accordingly. Dolls should be different, whether in terms of their faces, height or clothing, to minimize confusion issues. Clothing may vary according to the wishes of the patient or be supplemented with appropriate accessories such as a cap, socks, gloves, boots, blankets, and the like. We try to keep them clean. With doll therapy, we begin slowly and gradually to avoid problems that may be expressed as negative behaviour on the part of the patient, or repulsion from therapy, or the therapist.

We leave the doll for a short time, it is not appropriate to leave it all day, because the feelings that we should re-find in a patient with dementia may be lost that way.

We give the doll to the patient in an unforced manner, in order for them to decide whether to pay attention or not. It is appropriate if we place it in a well-visible and easily accessible place, where it can be seen and asked about or taken. If the patient is immobile or has a bad eyesight, we take the doll in our arms, sit down near them and start talking about it and talking to it. We monitor the patient's responses carefully, and when they show interest, we give it to them. Women and men may equally be interested in the doll, we do not discourage them from being so. When the patient communicates with their doll, we monitor and listen carefully to how they address her. We make sure we use their form of address to reassure them that we perceive it in the same way they do.

Some patients think the doll is their baby and they expect emotions and surprises, in which case we only leave it only for a short time. We take it only with their permission, with a logical explanation and detailed descriptions of where we are taking it and when we will return it. We do not leave the doll all day with the patient because it will stop interesting them. We never use the doll as something to negotiate or force the patient to do something. They can become emotionally attached to it, and so this can cause negative behaviour (anxiety, agitation, aggression). We can use it as an intermediary for other activities such as walks, talking and work.

There can also be undesirable situations in doll therapy. One of these is the recall of memories of a patient's negative life experiences. In such situations, the therapist must identify these events and pacify the patient appropriately.

Practical example:

We used doll therapy with a patient who had been diagnosed with Alzheimer's disease at a moderate level. She is aware of her illness, so she is reticent when talking about herself. From her past, she remembers most about the countryside near her home village. She answered every question asked after a pause and often indefinitely. She does not sufficiently show her emotions externally. She attributes her memory loss to age.

Sometimes she has hallucinations and attention disorders. Sometimes she talks nonsense. When communicating, she avoids direct gaze. We decided to use a therapeutic doll with the patient. We started in an unforced manner. One morning we brought the therapeutic doll that we held in our hands to the patient, and after a while the patient began to ask who it was, she wanted to take it in her arms. She began talking with her, singing her nursery rhymes. At other meetings she even named her after her daughter. We left the baby 1 or 2 hours, according to the interest shown. We did not use the baby every day so that the therapy did not become jaded but a pleasant emotional experience to revive the patient's psyche.

2.6 Ervin Böhm's psychobiographic model

Ervin Böhm's psychobiographic model is an internationally recognized nursing model and is currently the most widely used in German-speaking countries in the field of geriatric and gerontological psychiatric care. The model is aimed at supporting the ability to care for oneself, for old and confused people, and at ways to retain or restore this ability for as long as possible, by resurrecting the seniors' interest and reviving their psyche. In the psychobiographic model, one seeks to broaden the perspective on the patient—the senior, when care must become more tolerant and leave the 'caring mother' role. Previous methods of care, where the attending staff took care of all the tasks, did not reflect the retained skills and knowledge of the client, focused primarily on fulfilling needs, and created client dependence on care [25].

Böhm puts the following goals at the forefront of care:

a. reviving the human psyche,

b. reviving the interest of the carers, and

c. broadening the perception of social normality.

Reviving the Human Psyche—the ultimate goal of Böhm's care is to revive the soul of the old person, described as the human energy of the soul, the 'elan vital', which is the original source of our action and life-motivation. Revitalizing the interest of carers—reviving the professional interest of care providers can be achieved by increasing their expertise [25].

Böhm perceives his model of care as a complete systemic theory to supplement medical care. Regardless of whether a patient has organ damage, therapeutic treatment must be based on a thymopsychic biography, and must provide an improvement in their mental and physical well-being, even without psychopharmaceuticals [25].

If we focus on the medical and nursing diagnosis, then we take care of dementia, whereas if we focus on the biography of the client, we look after patient as a personality, so we see a person with his soul as a priority [26].

Practical demonstration:

A 67-year-old patient with a severe degree of Alzheimer's disease is hospitalized in the psychiatric ward for behavioural disorders, verbal and physical aggression, insomnia. At the age of 62 he had a stroke. The patient is disoriented with increased irritability and impulsiveness. Despite pharmacotherapy, the patient's behaviour is difficult to manage, and cooperation is limited. We focused on the biography of the patient, and together with the patient's wife, we looked for options that could influence patient behaviour and actions. The wife began talking about a special blanket that the patient had received as a wedding gift, having an emotional relationship, so we decided to use it during the hospitalization. The patient immediately recognized his blanket and expressed interest in it. The patient did not immediately reverse his behaviour, but with an empathic approach we managed to influence collaboration with the patient and mitigate aggressive behaviour.

Sometimes human desire is enough to achieve great goals.

3. The patient in the home environment

The family plays an essential role in the care of Alzheimer's disease. Most often it is the care provided by husbands, wives or children. In addition to the role of family members in the care of the sick, it is necessary to provide the carers with the support required. A common component of Alzheimer's disease is, in addition to behavioural disorders from disturbed cognition, various psychiatric symptoms. These are the main source of burden for carers and the most common cause of institutionalization of the sick. Problem behaviour by a sick person is often an effort to express or demonstrate their need. It arises as a result of the lack of consistency between the patient's needs and the ability of the environment to meet these needs. It may be a consequence of boredom or fatigue or the consequence of a psychiatric disorder. It is only a symptom of dementia, not deliberate or a bad intention. If we learn to recognize the needs of the sick, to satisfy them, then we can prevent these difficulties. Most often, this includes non-cooperation with care, restlessness, aggressive behaviour, wandering, getting lost and sleeping disorders [10].

3.1 Burden on the carer

The treatment of Alzheimer's disease stands on two pillars, but some authors add a third pillar, namely caring for the carer.

Nursing care provided in the home social environment is a historically proven form of effective care for an individual, family or community. It has a series of benefits for the care recipient themselves. The management of nursing care in the natural social environment varies in the individual countries of the European region, depending on historical development, the educational system, the financial possibilities and the requirements of society [27].

The family is the simplest, best and at the same time the most important source of support in old age and aging.

The family is the guarantor of the interconnection and continuity of individual generations and, under optimal functioning, forms an irreplaceable environment of mutual assistance, support and understanding for all its members, despite the intergenerational differences [28].

A home carer who provides care to a family member has an important place in the social and healthcare system. A home carer is a person who helps meet the needs of their family member—the person cared for. They also carry out activities that the patient would perform themselves if they had enough strength, will or the necessary knowledge [29].

The carer's role in the care of a sick person with dementia is a key factor. The work of caring for an elderly person is a task requiring a great deal of patience, empathy and sensitivity; it cannot be compared to normal work, especially if they do not feel satisfaction. Being the carer of an older person is to take on the responsibility of another person and includes the overall care for the person cared for. The carer must perform their duties extremely conscientiously and must think primarily of the welfare of the other person.

People who have to take care of the sick are exposed to many negative influences, because care is physically and mentally strenuous. Families often go through financial problems. The carer often loses the option of leaving the sufferer and it completely alters their rhythm of life. They may have problems at work, or have to leave employment. In addition to the above-mentioned negatives, they often feel helpless because they cannot help as they would wish, because the medical and nursing options are limited.

The perceived burden on the carer may be physical, psychological, social and financial. It can be a burden in areas such as free time, obligations towards one's own family, employment, but also relationships with others [29].

Counselling, self-help groups and nursing education programs are proven to de-institutionalize the patient, improve their quality of life and the satisfaction of family members and those affected by dementia [3].

In 2012, we conducted research aimed at identifying the extent and nature of the burden on people caring for relatives with Alzheimer's disease in the home environment. As a method for collecting empirical data, a valid, reliable questionnaire, The Zarit Caregiver Burden Interview, was used. The sample group consisted of 50 respondents, family carers for people with Alzheimer's disease. The results of the survey concurred with the results of several studies confirming that dependence of the patient on one caregiver is the most important factor affecting the caregiver's subjective burden.

4. Discussion

Caring for a patient with dementia is demanding, whether in the form of home or institutionalized care. Many experts have devoted large periods of their professional lives to studying care for patients with dementia, summarizing their knowledge and practical experience in theses as stated in the previous section. If we are concerned with the question of why the area of care for people with dementia is interesting for us, the answer is clear. Where pharmacological treatment is unsatisfactory and the actions and behaviour of the patient are impossible to control or predict, we search for opportunities to activate, stimulate, calm and fill time with meaningful activities. Doing nothing, lying in bed, wandering, negative moods and aggressive behaviour aggravate the overall condition of the patient and accelerate the progression of the disease. In addition to these important facts, it is important to remember the inability of a family carer or professional carer in institutionalized care to reverse this negative situation and do something extra for the sufferer. This is exactly how we see non-pharmacological approaches, which are based on a deep human principle. The experience of other professionals is extremely beneficial to those whom can be helped by these approaches to manage the actions and behaviour of patients and to arouse their interest. When working with relatives, we were deeply impressed by the approach of a daughter who was caring for her mother with Alzheimer's disease in her home environment. To the question: 'Why don't you put your mother in an old people's home, she doesn't know who you are anyway?' the daughter of the patient said, 'But *I* know who *she* is, she's my mother...'. Not everything can be quantified, verified or proven, so we continue to find new opportunities to improve the care of patients with dementia. The family or professional carer is the person who knows the patient very closely and chooses the approach that suits a particular patient. The conclusions of the experts are advisory, and the patient determines what is best. That is why care for a given patient can only ever be highly individualized.

The first empirical research into using therapeutic dolls for Alzheimer's disease was carried out in England in 2006. Later, further studies were performed and these confirmed a reduction in negative behaviour and wandering in patients, increased attention during contact with other people, increased food intake and improved mood [30].

Feil and de Klerk-Rubin proved their positive reactions by disoriented seniors.

If staff can create an atmosphere without conflict for their patients, and without the feeling that each thing has to be 'fought for' it means a lot to them. Another benefit to the patient is undoubtedly the fact that validation treats each person as a unique personality and respects them exactly as they are. This aspect applies in all spheres of the lives of seniors, starting with how they are spoken to [20].

Based on our findings, we can assume that the use of the psychobiographic model helps alleviate negative psychological phenomena, which is consistent with E. Böhm's assertions, and therefore the closer we approach the client with structured care, the more we reduce the many conflicting and hectic situations that lead to regression and pathological changes in client behaviour. Many studies have shown that increasing emotional stability leads to improvement of cognitive functions and conversely, decreasing emotional stability increases the progression of the cognitive deficit [25].

5. Conclusion

Given the demographic evolution of the population, it is essential to focus on identifying risk factors, focusing on appropriate planning of health care at the primary secondary and tertiary level [3]. Until there is a drug available to eliminate the cause of the disease, we rely on current therapeutic procedures, including pharmacological and non-pharmacological treatment and in the state of dependence not excluding care for the carer.

Acknowledgements

I thank to the Mgr. Adriana Gmitterová director of non-profit organization S.O.S. n.o., and to the Social services centre in Kruzľov for cooperation and creation of conditions for working with seniors.

Conflict of interest

The authors report no conflict of interest.

Author details

Terezia Fertalova* and Iveta Ondriova
Department of Nursing, University of Presov, Presov, Slovak Republic

*Address all correspondence to: terezia.fertalova@unipo.sk

References

[1] Holmerová I, Jarolímová E, Nováková H. Alzheimer's Disease in the Family. 1st ed. Prague: Pfizer; 2008. p. 116s

[2] Pidrman V. Dementia. 1st ed. Prague: Grada; 2007. 183 p. DOI: 978-80-247-1490-5

[3] Holmerová I, Jarolímová E, Suchá J. Care for a Patient with a Cognitive Disorder [Internet]. 2007. Available from: https://www.google.sk/url?sa=t&rct=j&q=&esrc=s&source=web&cd=1&ved=0ahUKEwiws42AzpzLAhWsE5oKHd3sCrMQFggbMAA&url=http%3A%2F%2Fwww.geriatrie.cz%2Fdokumenty%2FPece_o_pacienty_s_kognitivni_poruchou_1.pdf&usg=AFQjCNG6fRHU1_wbH9sRs1S8qaZdu21bpw&cad=rja [Accessed: Feb 22, 2016]

[4] Křížová J, Křemen J, Kotrlíková E, Svačina Š, et al. Enteral and Parenteral Nutrition. 2nd ed. Mladá fronta: Prague; 2014. 141 p. ISBN: 978-80-204-3326-8

[5] Forgáčová Ľ. Effect of nutrition supplements on cognitive functions: Knowledge from epidemiological and clinical studies. Praktické lekárnictvo. 2011;**1**(3):117-121. DOI: 1338-3132

[6] Poulose SM, Miller MG, Shukitt-Hale B. Role of Walnuts in Maintaining Brain Health with Age [Internet]. 2014. Available from: https://www.ncbi.nlm.nih.gov/pubmed/24500933 [Accessed: Dec 11, 2018]

[7] Herrmann N, Harimoto T, Balshaw R, Lanctôt KL. Risk Factors for Progression of Alzheimer Disease in a Canadian Population: The Canadian Outcomes Study in Dementia (COSID) [Internet]. 2015. Available from: http://search.proquest.com/docview/1674234502/B5AB8B90FB84E4FPQ/8?accountid=14716 [Accessed: Feb 22, 2016]

[8] Lairová S. Training of Memory. 3rd ed. Prague: Portál; 2011. 149 p. DOI: 978-80-7367-902-6

[9] Poledníková Ľ. Geriatric and Gerontological Nursing. 1st ed. Martin: Osveta; 2006. 216 p. DOI: 80-8063-208-1

[10] Jirák R, Holmerová I, Borzová C, et al. Dementia and Other Memory Disorders. 1st ed. Prague: Grada; 2009. 176 p. DOI: 978-80-247-2454-6

[11] Sheardová K. Alzheimer Disease and the Engagement of Informal Carers in a Fight for the Quality of Life [Internet]. 2010. Available from: http://www.neurologiepropraxi.cz/artkey/neu-201003-0008_Alzheimerova_nemoc_a_zapojeni_pecovatele_do_boje_o_kvalitu_zivota.php [Accessed: Feb 22, 2016]

[12] Suchá J. Train your Memory. 1st ed. Prague: Portál; 2010. 216 p. DOI: 978-80-7367-791-6

[13] Klímová E, Magurová D, et al. Theory and Practice in the Care of Patients with Alzheimer's Disease. 1st ed. Prešov: Univesity of Prešov; 2013. 235 p. DOI: 978-80-555-0936-5

[14] Fertaľová T, Ondriová I, Hadašová L. Treatment options of alzheimer's disease. Česká a slovenská psychiatrie. 2017;**113**(3):119-122. DOI: 1212-0383

[15] Tokovská M. Snoezelen as a leisure activity for seniors with dementia. Efeta. 2011;**21**(1):22-24. DOI: 1335-1397

[16] Janečková H, Vacková M. Reminiscence—Use Memories when Working with Seniors. 1st ed. Prague: Portál; 2010. 152 p. DOI: 978-80-7367-581-3

[17] Holmerová I, Janečková H, Vaňková H, Veleta P. Non-pharmacological

methods in the management of dementia and practical aspects of care. Psychiatria pre prax. 2005;**6**(4):175-178. DOI: 1335-9584

[18] Holmerová I. Care for a Patient with a Cognitive Disorder. 1st ed. Prague: Czech Alzheimer Society; 2009. 299 p. DOI: 978-80-86541-28-0

[19] Tavel P. Validation Therapy [Internet]. 2014. Available from: http://www.ostium.sk/sk/validacna-terapia/ [Accessed: Feb 19, 2016]

[20] Feil N, de Klerk-Rubin V. Validation. In: A Way to Understand Disoriented Old People. 9th ed. München: Ernst Reinhardt Verlag; 2010. DOI: 3-497-02156-7

[21] Feil N, de Klerk-Rubin V. Validation. In: The Way to Understand Old Disoriented People. 1st ed. Bratislava: Terapeutika; 2015. DOI: 978-80-971766-1-7

[22] Pokorná A, Sukupová M. Naomi Feil Validation® in Geriatric Care [Internet]. 2014. Available from: http://casopis-zsfju.zsf.jcu.cz/kontakt/clanky/1~2014/1109-ivalidace-podle-naomi-feil%C2%AE-i-v-geriatricke-peci [Accessed: Dec 12, 2018]

[23] Tavel P. Psychological Problems in the Old Age. 1st ed. Martin: Schola Philosophica; 2009. 279 p. DOI: 978-80-969823-7-0

[24] Braden BA, Gaspar PM. Implementation of a Baby Doll Therapy Protocol for People with Dementia (Inovative Practice) [Internet]. 2014. Available from: http://www.ncbi.nlm.nih.gov/pubmed/25432935 [Accessed: Feb 29, 2016]

[25] Procházková E. Work with Biography and Care Plans. 1st ed. Prague: Mladá fronta; 2014. 133 p. DOI: 978-80-204-3186-8

[26] Böhm E. Psychobiographisches Pflegemodell nach Böhm. 4st ed. Wien-München-Bern: Wilhelm Maudrich GmbH & Co KG; 2009. 289 p. DOI: 9783851759112

[27] Padyšáková H, Kovácsová O. Management of Home Nursing Care [Internet]. 2010. Available from: http://www.osetrovatelsky.herba.sk/index.php/rok-2010/34-6-2010/199-manazment-domacej-osetrovatelskej-starostlivosti [Accessed: Oct 17, 2016]

[28] Selická D, Solčianska A. Intergenerational Impact of Family Relationships, Conflicts and Solidarity in the Family. 1st ed. Nitra: UKF; 2013. 146 p. DOI: 978-80558-0435-4

[29] Tabáková M, Václavíková P. Burden in Family Caregiver [Internet]. 2008. Available from: https://profeseonline.upol.cz/pdfs/pol/2008/02/03.pdf [Accessed: May 12, 2017]

[30] Mitchell G, Temleton M. Enthical Considerations of Doll Therapy for People with Dementia [Internet]. 2014. Available from: http://www.pulib.sk:2172/ehost/pdfviewer/pdfviewer?vid=5&sid=ea6c5574-1d30-49d4-9d42-dbedcc59a32e%40sessionmgr112hid=109 [Accessed: Jan 26, 2015]

Chapter 6

Healthcare Models in Alzheimer's Disease

Francisco Javier Garzón-Maldonado and María Dolores Martinez-Valle Torres

Abstract

Alzheimer's disease is currently a health care problem and in the future, when we have effective treatments, it will become a public health priority. Health systems should adapt to this situation. New technologies are tools that can improve healthcare and lower costs. The mobile phone with call o video call conference is going to suppose a radical change in the control of these patients. The telephone assistance to patient or relatives is very satisfactory for both due to the rapidity in the response to their problem and the comfort with which they are attended to. Also the health system reduces the costs of face-to-face consultation.
In addition, this telemedicine could be applied for cognitive stimulation, with specific programs for each patient and for the follow-up of patients in their homes, delaying their entry into residences. The objective is to turn the patients and their caregiver into cotherapists together with the nurse and the physician, in the follow-up of Alzheimer's disease.

Keywords: healthcare, Alzheimer's disease

1. Alzheimer's disease: public health priority

Alzheimer's disease (AD) is a degenerative disease produced by the accumulation of beta-amyloid and tau protein in the brain. From the clinical point of view, it is characterized by a prodromal phase with mild cognitive impairment, which is followed by the dementia phase [1].

Early dementia screening by a primary care physician should be completed once a patient or a knowledgeable informant has noticed decline in memory or difficulty [2]. Screening is not indicated at the general population level [3, 4], because currently there are no specific treatments to block the progression of cognitive decline in AD and other neurocognitive dementias. Is very important reasons from a patient's social and personal perspective that an early diagnosis is important as Alzheimer's disease is a terminal illness; you can minimize some of the effects if you understand the disease and know what to do [5]. Numerous screening tests are available for confirmed cognitive impairment, and laboratory tests and imaging studies should be obtained to rule out reversible etiologies. If patients meet diagnostic criteria for AD, clinicians should educate patients and caregivers on the expected course and help them complete advance directives. Troublesome behaviors should be managed with nonpharmacotherapeutic measures first. Drugs for improving cognition can be prescribed but do not prevent disease progression [6]. Patients with advanced illness need end of life care (EoLC) with adequate pain control and palliative care interventions to shorten their hospital stay. Bamford et al. [7] take seven factors influencing good EoLC for people with dementia (**Table 1**). By incorporating stakeholders' perspectives and preferences when planning and developing coordinating interventions, we may increase the likelihood of successful implementation and patient benefits [8].

In 1984, the National Institute of Neurological and Communicative Disorders and Stroke and the Alzheimer's Disease and Related Disorders Association (NINCDS-ADRA) developed the first diagnostic criteria for Alzheimer's dementia [9]. In 2011, the National Institute of Aging/Alzheimer's Association (NIA-AA) revised these criteria including two new phases of the disease and introduced the utilization of biomarkers in research. Firstly, the introduction of the use of biomarkers would aim to detect pathological changes of AD before the onset of cognitive symptoms—"the preclinical phase" [10]. Secondly, the introduction of a mildly symptomatic but not dementia phase, which defines the onset of mild cognitive symptoms, was introduced. Clinical biomarkers such as deposition of Aβ seen on PET imaging were introduced to increase the clinical likelihood of diagnosis of AD on the presentation of mild cognitive impairment (MCI) however, these are yet to be utilized for routine clinical use [11]. In 2014, the International Working Group updated their clinical entity of prodromal AD by introducing improved biomarkers for AD and defining a criteria for atypical and non-AD dementia [12]. And finally, the diagnostic standard for dementia is the *Diagnostic and Statistical Manual of Mental Disorders, Fifth Edition* (*DSM-5*). *DSM-5* recognizes two cognitive syndromes: major neurocognitive impairment and mild neurocognitive impairment. The diagnosis of major neurocognitive impairment requires objective cognitive

Summary of the seven factors influencing good EoLC for people with dementia

Undertaking timely planning discussions to ensure plans are discussed when the person with dementia has capacity and that they are documented and disseminated as appropriate.
Recognising end of life and providing supportive care to ensure effective management of key symptoms (e.g. pain, anxiety and nausea), and minimise distress by providing comfort in a familiar environment.
Co-ordination and continuity of care includes liaison between day and night staff in services and having established links with local services (e.g. hospices), particularly for support out of hours.
Working effectively with primary care can be facilitated by having a named liaison person in the practice. For care homes, liaison can be improved by regular routine visits and limiting the number of general practices with which residents are registered.
Managing hospitalisation includes avoiding unnecessary admissions by appropriate out-of-hours support and documentation of wishes and preferences. It also involves managing admission and discharge effectively where hospitalisation is necessary.
Continuing care after death to enable family members to be supported by known members of staff who cared for the person with dementia at the end of life. This continuity of care is valued by family members.
Valuing staff and ongoing learning facilitates staff retention and results in a more skilled and knowledgeable workforce. Stable staff teams are more able to detect emotional vulnerability in their colleagues and ensure timely and appropriate support.

Table 1.
Summary of the seven factors influencing good EoLC for people with dementia.

decline that is severe enough to interfere with activities of daily living and is not caused by delirium or another neurologic, medical, or psychiatric disorder [13].

The socio-health needs of dementias are similar, regardless of their etiology, although there are some peculiarities that characterize each of them like hallucinations in dementia by Lewy bodies, behavioral problems in frontotemporal dementia, and social and emotional level of loneliness, which is higher in Korsakoff syndrome [14]. This social and emotional loneliness is more frequent and earlier income in a residence of the patients with Korsakoff syndrome [15].

In 2010, annual healthcare costs attributable to dementia were between $41,000 and $56,000 per person [16]. About three quarters of these costs are from institutional and home-based long-term care. Although these estimates place a monetary value on informal care provided by family members and friends, they do not account for the substantial non-monetary costs to caregivers in terms of negative consequences to social, physical, and psychological well-being [17]. If we can delay dependency and institutionalization, by even a couple of years, it has the potential to save hundreds of billions in direct healthcare costs and even more in terms of improved well-being for caregivers.

The AD from the clinical point of view is today a public health problem recognized by the WHO [18], because it is a very frequent disease. It is estimated that 46.8 million people live with dementia in the world in 2015. This number is expected to double every 20 years, reaching 74.7 million in 2030 and 131.5 million in 2050. This translates to approximately two new cases per 1000 people age 65–74, 13 new cases per 1000 people age 75–84, and 39 new cases per 1000 people age 85 and older, and the greatest risk factor by far is aging [19–21]. It is also a disease with great impact on the health of the patient, who becomes totally dependent, and the family environment, for their involvement in the care from the physical and psychological point of view. On average, a person with Alzheimer's disease will spend more years (40% of the total number of years with Alzheimer's) in the most severe stage of the disease than in any other stages. However, currently, and from an epidemiological point of view, it is not a priority in health, given that although we have a screening test for the population, we do not have a drug with the potential to significantly modify the natural course of the disease. The quality of care received by a person with dementia positively is critical to the physical and mental health of the person with dementia [22]. It is a challenge for socio-health systems to determine what needs should be provided and financed.

2. Needs and demands socio-health of the patients

Dementia is a chronic and progressive disease, with an average survival of more than 10 years. Patient and the family environment with this disease go through different phases that have different needs and demands. The needs are determined by the interventions that have shown efficacy through scientific studies, while the demands are determined mainly by sociocultural factors. A clear example of this is that new generations accept new technologies much better than previous generations [23]. Any socio-health system should try to provide its patients and caregivers with those needs and demands as efficiently as possible (actions with studies that demonstrate their effectiveness and that are viable from the economic point of view). In general, caregivers claim and request less formal attention than in other pathologies [24]. Each patient with dementia and its family have different characteristics and needs that require individual attention [25]. The NICE guide recommends periodic evaluation and caregiver programs, including telephone or Internet support. Such supportive interventions could be effective both preventive and therapeutic of the consequences of the burden [26]. The unmet needs may be higher in caregivers with lower education and individuals with early-stage dementia and low-income. The identifying and treating symptoms of depression in patients with dementia and caregivers are necessary for them to know their other unmet needs [27].

Socio-sanitary assistance to dementia has the highest degree of complexity, comparable to multi-pathological patients, according to the categorization of chronic patients adopted by the Department of Health of the United Kingdom, the approach of the Kaiser Permanente. These patients require a comprehensive and continuous treatment, which must be based on the coordination of healthcare and social assistance, as well as between the different levels of care (primary care and specialized care). And more specifically in health care, the link between the specialist physician and the case management nurse of the unit with primary care is key, so that this assistance has a versatility that allows ensuring adequate care more appropriate [28].

The personalized care plan focuses on the patient with the disease but involves the entire family environment of the patient, understanding this environment widely, including friends and volunteers, among others.

The aim of the personalized care plan are: (1) promotion of the autonomy of the patient with activation and self-management of care and improvement of their quality of life; (2) pharmacotherapeutic optimization at all times during the disease; (3) prevent complications, cognitive and functional impairment, and ultimately dependence; (4) integral assessment of the patient from a biomedical or clinical, psychological, functional and socio-family point of view; (5) establishment of a prognosis in each phase of the disease; (6) establish advance planning of decisions.

The needs or demands of patients and caregivers with dementia are typified and all socio-health systems establish different socio-sanitary responses to similar pathologies [26, 29, 30]. However, this assistance must be individualized in each specific user always, considering it as a biopsychosocial organism, with its particular desires and preferences. Therefore, assistance to users with AD must be protocolized in a multidisciplinary way and provided individually to each patient and caregiver.

In spite of the increase of the income in residences in the last years, the family environment is the therapeutic reference that is more effective, efficient, and very difficult to substitute for the emotional implications that it has. And above all, it is preferred by most patients with dementia [31–33]. The competence of caregivers is essential for the life quality of patient with dementia, and multicomponent interventions may be appropriate for nurses to practice [34].

3. Social sanitary assistance management tools

We must overcome health care in the terms of first-visit patients and regulated reviews (at 3, 6, 9, or 12 months) and use management tools that use information and communication technologies to satisfy the needs and demands, avoiding referrals, appointments, and bureaucratic reviews.

Among the emerging management tools in recent years that are most useful are:

1. Caregivers: we have to pay much more attention to the caregiver or caregivers and use them as cotherapists, throughout the process, especially in the final phase [35].

2. Case management nurse [36, 37]: together with the medical specialist or general practitioner who is, usually, the axis around which health care is provided. The case management nurse coordinates all the actions of the patient and their

family. The liaison nurse of the dementia unit, within a neurology service, was the axis around which social-health assistance was established. In our study [37], the case management nurse of the dementia unit, was the axis around which social-health assistance was established.

3. Coordination with de Alzheimer's association using their ability to bring together the patient and the family environment, using their infrastructures and volunteering to monitor users [38, 39].

4. Digital clinical history: access to the digital clinical history instantly, from any terminal of the health system (both primary care and specialized care), allows to efficiently solve healthcare problems in relation to the patient without the inconvenience of having to travel or the delay of having to wait for an appointment.

5. Prescription on line: also accessible from any terminal of the health system. It allows to see the medication prescribed by any doctor to the patient. It has the potential to establish alerts, system of interactions and allergies, and maximum duration of treatments, among others.

6. Telecare: At the beginning it arose to solve the problems of accessibility in remote areas and sanitary underfunded, allowed accessibility by spacing distances. Subsequently, it was considered that telemedicine contributed essential quality by facilitating the continuity of care, and recently it is considered an efficient and essential tool in the organization of health care. The application of technology in health has become a strategic objective to address the demographic challenge and allow "aging at home."

The modalities of telecare can be very diverse, and the telemedicine projects of attention to users with dementia performed include [1] support for patients so that they can continue to live independently; [2] support services for informal caregivers through "online" training, video conferencing with professionals, telealarm with videoconference, and cognitive stimulation; [3] networks for patient and caregivers; [4] monitoring of the state of the patient, personalized intervention, and adaptive care; [5] platform that integrates smart home technologies, with sensors and interoperability with professionals and institutions; and [6] computer programs to caregivers to improve their overload, mainly emotional.

The main problems of this technology are the risks of privacy in relation to data protection and health care. Other issues technological aspects that are solved with the progress of technology: complexity of use, cost of acquisition and technical failures.

The main resistance for its establishment is given by the three protagonists of the assistance: patients and caregivers, professionals, and mainly the managers of the health administration [40].

These tools used by each socio-health system according to their possibilities allow a better assistance to patients and caregivers.

4. Health model units of cognitive disorder and conduct

Dementia is the paradigm of disease that practically in its entirety is diagnosed and/or followed by the national health systems (public and free). It is a disease that does not start abruptly and for which medicines are expensive. Patient assistance involves the neurologists and other specialists who directly assist patients with neurological problems. The growing complexity of neurology in general, as a specialty, with the improvement of diagnostic methods as well as therapeutic interventions, means that the assistance provided by a neurologist or psychiatrist or geriatrist is greater.

The guiding principles of the assistance in the unit of memory are [1] universality and equality; [2] integrality and transversality, with coordination of all the members; and [3] efficiency and sustainability. This unit must be endowed with the human and material resources to meet its objectives [41, 42].

- Comprehensive care for affected people and support for caregivers in all phases of dementia.

- Information, training, and advice to affected people, caregivers, associations, and professionals involved in dementia assistance.

- Sensitization of public opinion, institutions, entities, and media.

- Adequacy of health and social resources, as well as the establishment of protocols and joint procedures.

- Promotion of volunteering and promotion of associations.

- Promote lines of research and intervention.

To fulfill these objectives, within the unit there should be another specialist doctor (neurologist, psychiatrist, and geriatrist), nurse manager of hospital cases, clinical psychologist or neuropsychologist, and social worker.

In primary care, it should consist of a family doctor and nurse who manages primary care cases and social work. The coordination and communication between these professionals is key in dementia care process.

To carry out all its objectives, you should use the tools, mainly new technologies, of which the health system has: digital clinical history, prescription "online," and telecare.

Key aspects in the operation of the unit that should be considered:

1. Management of communication at all levels: horizontal internal, between the members of the unit among themselves and with the other professionals of the organization; internal vertical, with the address of the hospital and primary care center; external with patients and relatives, with associations of relatives of patients and with society in general [43].

2. Control of the satisfaction of all those who participate in the unit: patients and relatives, professionals, and the administration in relation to the activities developed in relation to the healthcare process.

3. Establish indicators of care process, health outcomes, and specific situations: all this must be reflected in an annual report of the unit, which includes all the activity of the unit carried out, mainly in the care, research, and teaching areas.

The personalized attention in the chronic disease improves the indicators of physical and psychological health, as well as the ability to manage the disease with respect to usual care. The differences increase when they are more complete and more intense and integrated into the routine. Care with a more personalized and graduated approach allows to maintain the autonomy and integration of the patient in his environment [44, 45]. The coordination at the health level between primary and specialized care, with a social worker and in association with Alzheimer's patients' relatives, all tools being available (telephone, email, digital medical record, prescription "online"), is key for the success in monitoring patients and caregivers [37].

5. Future perspectives

The optimism generated by recent and anticipated developments in the understanding and treatment of Alzheimer's disease presents a great opportunity to innovate and adapt our services to incorporate the next exciting development in the field of dementia [46]. Almost 100 treatments are currently being investigated, often targeting individuals earlier in the disease process, and a very promising phase II work has been published about the antibody aducanumab [47]. Today, health services in Europe would not be prepared to treat patients with Alzheimer's disease that are subsidized by an effective treatment [48]. It seems likely that interventions will be available in the near future for people diagnosed with prodromal dementia. This would fundamentally transform how the Alzheimer's disease is perceived, diagnosed, and managed.

There are two key points: [1] equity in access of patients and caregivers and [2] specific preparation of professionals. There will be a need for substantial education and training for primary and secondary care professionals about new disease-modifying treatment for Alzheimer's disease. In primary care this would need to focus on early symptoms and risk factors. In secondary care it would cover the safe and effective use of biomarkers. A reconfigured service would require seamless collaboration between disciplines, patient groups, and specialties in order to expand the dementia-focused clinical services to include an Alzheimer's disease service. While many people currently present with moderate or severe dementia, in the future, hopefully the majority of people will be diagnosed much earlier, even in the prodromal/preclinical stages. A distinct approach for the preclinical, prodromal, and dementia stages of Alzheimer's disease would be necessary.

- Healthcare systems will need to identify and engage with prodromal populations who might benefit from such interventions. These people may not be in contact with health services or, if they are, this will not be because of Alzheimer's disease.

- Realistic planning is needed now to direct the evolution of services to optimize appropriate patient access and prepare protocols for phase IV testing of these treatments to inform real-world practice and commissioning decisions.

Although in the near future we will have treatment for Alzheimer's disease, the social-health system will have to continue providing assistance in stages of dementia, in an integral and personalized way, adapting to the specific needs of each case that is determined by the type of dementia (frontotemporal, dementia by bodies of Lewy, and Korsakoff syndrome), characteristics of the patient, or caregiver environment.

Author details

Francisco Javier Garzón-Maldonado[1] and María Dolores Martinez-Valle Torres[2*]

1 Hospital Universitario Virgen de la Victoria, Málaga, Spain

2 Hospital Universitario San Cecilio, Granada, Spain

*Address all correspondence to: mariad.martinezvalle.sspa@juntadeandalucia.es

References

[1] Lane CA, Hardy J, Schott JM. Alzheimer's disease. European Journal of Neurology. 2018;**25**(1):59-70

[2] Panegyres PK, Berry R, Burchell J. Early dementia screening. Diagnostics (Basel). 2016;**6**(1):1-13. DOI:10.3390/diagnostics6010006

[3] Lliffe S, Manthorpe J. The hazards of early recognition of dementia: A risk assessment. Aging & Mental Health. 2004;**8**:99-105

[4] Erlangsen A, Zarit SH, Conwell Y. Hospital-diagnosed dementia and suicide: A longitudinal study using prospective, nationwide register data. The American Journal of Geriatric Psychiatry. 2008;**16**(3):220-228

[5] Okie S. Confronting Alzheimer's disease. The New England Journal of Medicine. 2011;**365**(12):1069-1072

[6] Kemle K, Ackermann RJ. Issues in geriatric care: Alzheimer disease. FP Essentials. 2018;**468**:26-34

[7] Bamford C, Lee R, McLellan E, Poole M, Harrison-Dening K, Hughes J, et al. What enables good end of life care for people with dementia? A multi-method qualitative study with key stakeholders. BMC Geriatrics. 2018;**18**(1):302

[8] Backhouse A, Richards DA, McCabe R, Watkins R, Dickens C. Stakeholders perspectives on the key components of community-based interventions coordinating care in dementia: A qualitative systematic review. BMC Health Services Research. 2017;**17**(1):767

[9] McKhann G, Drachman D, Folstein M, Katzman R, Price D, Stadlan EM. sClinical diagnosis of Alzheimer's disease: Report of the NINCDS-ADRDA Work Group under the auspices of Department of Health and Human Services Task Force on Alzheimer's Disease. Neurology. 1984;**34**(7):939-944

[10] Sperling RA, Aisen PS, Beckett LA, Bennett DA, Craft S, Fagan AM, et al. Toward defining the preclinical stages of Alzheimer's disease: Recommendations from the National Institute on Aging-Alzheimer's Association workgroups on diagnostic guidelines for Alzheimer's disease. Alzheimer's & Dementia. 2011;**7**(3):280-292

[11] Albert MS, DeKosky ST, Dickson D, Dubois B, Feldman HH, Fox NC, et al. The diagnosis of mild cognitive impairment due to Alzheimer's disease: Recommendations from the National Institute on Aging-Alzheimer's Association workgroups on diagnostic guidelines for Alzheimer's disease. Alzheimer's & Dementia. 2011;**7**(3):270-279

[12] Dubois B, Feldman HH, Jacova C, Cummings JL, Dekosky ST, Barberger-Gateau P, et al. Revising the definition of Alzheimer's disease: A new lexicon. Lancet Neurology. 2010;**9**:1118-1127

[13] American Psychiatric Association. Diagnostic and Statistical Manual of Mental Disorders, Fifth Edition, DSM-5. Arlington, VA: American Psychiatric Association; 2013

[14] Oudman E, van Dam M, Postma A. Social and emotional loneliness in Korsakoff's syndrome. Cognitive Neuropsychiatry. 2018;**23**(5):307-320

[15] Oudman E, Wijnia JW. Evolution of quality of life in patients with Korsakoff's syndrome in a long-term care facility. International Psychogeriatrics. 2014;**26**(12):2073-2079

[16] Hurd MD, Martorell P, Langa KM. Monetary costs of dementia in the United States. New England Journal of Medicine. 2013;**369**:489-490

[17] Etters L, Goodall D, Harrison BE. Caregiver burden among dementia

patient caregivers: A review of the literature. Journal of the American Academy of Nurse Practitioners. 2008;**20**(8):423-428

[18] Wortmann M. Dementia: A global health priority-highlights from an ADI and world health organization report. Alzheimer's research and therapy. 2012;**4**:40. https://doi.org/10.1186/alzrt143

[19] 2015Alzheimer's disease facts and figures. Alzheimer's & Dementia. 2015;**11**(3):332-384

[20] Niu H, Alvarez-Alvarez I, Guillen-Grima F, Aguinaga-Ontoso I. Prevalence and incidence of Alzheimer's disease in Europe: A meta-analysis. Neurología. 2017;**32**(8):523-532

[21] Esiri MM, Chance SA. Cognitive reserve, cortical plasticity and resistance to Alzheimer's disease. Alzheimer's Research & Therapy. 2012;**4**(2):7

[22] World Alzheimer's Report 2009. London: Alzheimer's Disease International; 2009

[23] Garzon-Maldonado FJ, Gutierrez-Bedmar M, Garcia-Casares N, Perez-Errazquin F, Gallardo-Tur A, Martinez-Valle Torres MD. Health-related quality of life in caregivers of patients with Alzheimer's disease. Neurología. 2017;**32**(8):508-515

[24] Bakker C, de Vugt ME, van Vliet D, Verhey FR, Pijnenburg YA, Vernooij-Dassen MJ, et al. The use of formal and informal care in early onset dementia: Results from the NeedYD study. The American Journal of Geriatric Psychiatry. 2013;**21**(1):37-45

[25] Charlesworth G, Shepstone L, Wilson E, Thalanany M, Mugford M, Poland F. Does befriending by trained lay workers improve psychological well-being and quality of life for carers of people with dementia, and at what cost? A randomised controlled trial. Health Technology Assessment. 2008; **12**(4):1-78, iii, v-ix

[26] National Collaborating Centre for Mental H. National Institute for Health and Clinical Excellence: Guidance. Dementia: A NICE-SCIE Guideline on Supporting People with Dementia and Their Carers in Health and Social Care. Leicester (UK): British Psychological Society. The British Psychological Society & The Royal College of Psychiatrists; 2007

[27] Black BS, Johnston D, Rabins PV, Morrison A, Lyketsos C, Samus QM. Unmet needs of community-residing persons with dementia and their informal caregivers: Findings from the maximizing independence at home study. Journal of the American Geriatrics Society. 2013;**61**(12):2087-2095

[28] Dirección Regional de Desarrollo e Innovación en Cuidados. Manual jde la Gestion de Casos en Andalucia: Enfermeras Gestoras de Casos en Atención Primaria. Revisado Febrero de 2007

[29] Egdell V. Who cares? Managing obligation and responsability across the changing landscapes of informal dementia care. Ageing and Society. 2013;**33**(5):888-907

[30] Andalucía CdSJd. Proceso Asistencial Integrado Demencia. 2002. Available from: http://www.juntadeandalucia.es/salud/sites/csalud/contenidos/Informacion_General/p_3_p_3_procesos_asistenciales_integrados/pai/demencia_v3?perfil=org

[31] Carpentier N. Caregiver identity as a useful concept for understanding the linkage between formal and informal care systems: A case study. Sociology Mind. 2012;**2**(1):41-49

[32] Crellin NE, Orrell M, McDermott O, Charlesworth G. Self-efficacy and health-related quality of life in family carers of people with dementia: A

systematic review. Aging & Mental Health. 2014;**18**(8):954-969

[33] Donath C, Winkler A, Graessel E, Luttenberger K. Day care for dementia patients from a family caregiver's point of view: A questionnaire study on expected quality and predictors of utilisation—Part II. BMC Health Services Research. 2011;**11**:76

[34] Ying J, Wang Y, Zhang M, Wang S, Shi Y, Li H, et al. Effect of multicomponent interventions on competence of family caregivers of people with dementia: A systematic review. Journal of Clinical Nursing. 2018;**27**(9-10):1744-1758

[35] Practice guideline for the treatment of patients with Alzheimer's disease and other dementias of late life. American Psychiatric Association. The American Journal of Psychiatry. 1997;**154**(5 Suppl):1-39

[36] Dirección General de Asistencia Sanitaria. Dirección Regional de Desarrollo e Inovación en Cuidados. Manual de Gestión de Casos en Andalucia. Revisión Noviembre 2006

[37] Garzon-Maldonado FJ, Gutierrez-Bedmar M, Serrano-Castro V, Requena-Toro MV, Padilla-Romero L, Garcia-Casares N. An assessment of telephone assistance systems for caregivers of patients with Alzheimer's disease. Neurología. 2017;**32**(9):595-601

[38] Consejería de Salud Junta de Andalucía C. AL LADO. Itinerario de Atención Compartida de Demencias/Alzheimer. 2011. Available from: http://www.juntadeandalucia.es/salud/sites/csalud/contenidos/Informacion_General/c_3_c_1_vida_sana/dependencia/al_lado

[39] http://www.i2cat.net/es/proyectos/afa-connectalzheimer

[40] Christie HL, Bartels SL, Boots LMM, Tange HJ, Verhey FJJ, de Vugt ME. A systematic review on the implementation of eHealth interventions for informal caregivers of people with dementia. Internet Interventions. 2018;**13**:51-59

[41] Ministerio de Sanidad. Estrategia para el abordaje de la cronicidad en el Sistema Nacional de Salud. Madrid; 2012. Disponible en: http://publicacionesoficiales.boe.es

[42] Estrategia de Alzheimer de Andalucia. Junta de Andalucia. In: Consejeria de Salud. 2017 www.juntadeandalucia.es/salud

[43] Molinuevo JL, Peña-Casanova J. Guía oficial para la práctica clínica en demencias: Conceptos, criterios y recomendaciones 2009

[44] Pimouguet C, Bassi V, Somme D, Lavallart B, Helmer C, Dartigues JF. The 2008-2012 French Alzheimer plan: A unique opportunity for improving integrated care for dementia. Journal of Alzheimer's Disease. 2013;**34**(1):307-314

[45] Somme D, Corvol A, Couturier Y, Pimouguet C, Moreau O, Perivier S, et al. New professional field in France: Analysis of the training needs of case managers. Santé Publique. 2015; **27**(1 Suppl):S61-S66

[46] Ritchie CW, Russ TC, Banerjee S, Barber B, Boaden A, Fox NC, et al. The Edinburgh Consensus: Preparing for the advent of disease-modifying therapies for Alzheimer's disease. Alzheimer's Research & Therapy. 2017;**9**(1):85

[47] Sevigny J, Chiao P, Bussiere T, Weinreb PH, Williams L, Maier M, et al. The antibody aducanumab reduces Abeta plaques in Alzheimer's disease. Nature. 2016;**537**(7618):50-56

[48] The Lancet N. Will Europe be ready for the treatment of Alzheimer's disease? Lancet Neurology. 2018;**17**(12):1025

Chapter 7

An Examination of Factors Influencing Equitable Access to Dementia Care and Support Programs among Migrants and Refugees Living with Dementia: A Literature Review

Winnie Sun, Srija Biswas, Michelle Dacanay and Ping Zou

Abstract

Canada is working on improving the diagnosis and treatment of Canadians with cognitive impairment and promoting living well with dementia. Despite the availability of support network, Canadians living with dementia are identified to commonly experience social isolation and exclusion. This issue is particularly significant among migrants and refugees, for whom access to dementia care and support programs are found to be significantly less than the non-migrated Canadians. The purpose of this critical analysis is to examine the existing literature related to the sociocultural factors that contribute to the access of dementia care and support programs by persons with dementia. Specifically, a literature review was conducted to examine the barriers and facilitating factors that influence equitable access to dementia care and support programs among migrants and refugees. A thematic analysis was conducted to identify the following four major themes: (1) stigma, (2) culturally preferred coping strategies, (3) misconceptions regarding aging and dementia, and (4) language barriers.. This review identifies the need for future research to explore the key barriers faced by migrants and refugees with dementia in accessing timely and appropriate dementia care and support programs, as well as developing equitable programs and culturally sensitive services that adequately address their needs.

Keywords: literature review, migrants, immigrants, refugees, sociocultural barriers, access, dementia care

1. Introduction

1.1 Background

Dementia has been identified as one of the leading issues concerning people over the age of 65. A number of Canadians aged 40 and older living with Alzheimer's disease and other forms of dementia are expected to increase over time. In fact, this increase will be from about 395,000 in 2016 to 674,000 in 2031 [1]. In the Statistics Canada 2016 report, it estimated that 35.6 million global citizens were living with dementia and that the number is expected to double within the next 20 years [2]. When diagnosing an individual with dementia, physicians refer to the Diagnostic Manual of Mental Disorders (DSM) as a guide when determining whether the individual shows progressive tendencies of dementia [3]. The manual that is currently in practice is the DSM-5, which classifies dementia as a neurocognitive disorder. Generally, dementia is an umbrella term that encompasses a variety of symptoms related to the decline of cognitive function, which influences a person's ability to execute everyday activities [3]. In order to be diagnosed with dementia, one must meet certain criterions listed in the DSM-5 when determining major neurocognitive disorders such as (a) showing evidence of significant mental decline that interferes with mundane daily routines or (b) for milder cases showing signs of modest cognitive decline with only little interference of daily active living [4]. The DSM-5 criteria for tendencies of dementia include (1) cognitive changes, including new forgetfulness and difficulty finding words; (2) psychiatric symptoms, such as withdrawal or apathy, depression, and anxiety; (3) personality changes, such as blunting and disinterest and social withdrawal; (4) problem behaviors, such as wandering, agitation, and restlessness; and (5) changes in day-to-day functioning, including difficulty driving, getting lost, neglecting self-care, and difficulty handling money [3].

There are different forms of dementia due to variances in the distinct expression of symptoms in addition to structural brain abnormalities. One of the most common forms of dementia is Alzheimer's disease, followed closely then by vascular dementia [5]. Other known types of dementia include dementia with Lewy bodies (DLB) and frontotemporal dementia. Moreover, impaired mental functions that arise due to the neurodegenerative disease include memory, language and communication, judgment and reasoning, and attention span [3]. Even emotional control and social behavior and motivation are altered and may deteriorate as the disease progresses. Rates of dementia, including Alzheimer's disease and other forms of illness, are projected to increase continuously and double every 20 years [6]. It is estimated that in 2010, over 35 million people worldwide were living with dementia [7]. Dementia and Alzheimer's disease are considered as an abnormal process of aging. Common symptomology includes frequent memory loss and finding family members and friends unrecognizable [8]. It is believed that people first experience an asymptomatic period where neurodegenerative changes occur in the brain, while cognitive abilities remain stable. This preliminary phase occurs for a long duration and is followed by the progressive cognitive decline and the eventual, late-stage development of dementia [9].

Living with dementia means coping with the progressive loss of physical and mental abilities. It can have an overwhelming negative impact on the individual and those around them by progressively altering every part of their life until the individual becomes completely dependent on either their loved ones, paid caregivers, or a combination of both. Living with dementia imposes a large physical health, mental health, and economic burden on the patients, informal caregivers, and family member [10]. It can affect the patient in many ways starting from increased dependency on caregivers for daily life activities, inability to be engaged in activities that they were previously able to, leading to frustration and short-temperedness, depression and anxiety, confusion, and fear [11]. Regardless of the availability of a strong support network, people with dementia have been identified to commonly face isolation, loneliness, and social exclusion. In order to improve the quality of life of individuals living with dementia and their caregivers, Canada is implementing national strategies and community level actions to improve and strengthen their support network and with the aim of promoting living well with dementia [12]. Cultural diversity is one of the key characteristics that defines the current Canadian demographic shift. It is estimated that by 2031, visible minorities from multicultural backgrounds among whom majority have lived in Canada for less than 15 years will make up approximately 63% of the population in Toronto, the largest city in Canada [13]. Increasing the number of migrants will lead to an increasing number of persons with dementia from various cultural backgrounds. As the dementia community possesses increased cultural diversity, it is crucial to identify the relationship between sociocultural factors and access to support programs aimed at promoting living well with dementia [14, 15]. Similarly, refugee populations of every age group living in a foreign country often suffer from various challenges including language difficulties, acculturative stress, loneliness, and societal prejudice, leading to a depleted social network and barriers to accessing necessary services and supports [4]. In particular, a reduced level of participation is observed in dementia care and support programs among immigrants and refugees compared to their nonimmigrant counterparts [15]. There is a need to increase our understanding about the unique needs of the immigrants and refugees with dementia that would promote their timely and appropriate access to dementia support services in the community.

1.2 Objective

The purpose of this chapter is to review the existing literature related to the persons living with dementia who have migrated as a refugee or immigrant and to explore the sociocultural factors that contribute to the access to dementia care and support programs among these vulnerable populations. Our literature review will place special emphasis on the Southeast Asian population because the number of people living with dementia in the Asia Pacific region will triple between now and year 2050 with Alzheimer's disease being projected to rise by 300% among Southeast Asians, the highest projected rise among other ethnic groups [31].

This literature review aims at:

1. identifying the sociocultural factors influencing access to and participation in dementia care and support programs among migrants and refugees, with emphasis on Southeast Asian populations;

2. exploring knowledge gaps in the existing literature to identify further research opportunities in relation to improving access to dementia care and support programs for migrant and refugee populations.

2. Method

In order to address the above objectives, a literature review was conducted using a predetermined inclusion-exclusion criteria and search strategy as outlined below.

2.1 Inclusion and exclusion criteria

The search strategy for the literature review included journal articles and research papers that were published until May 2017. A preliminary search was conducted on this topic to determine the scope of the existing literature, which has revealed a lack of published research in the field of dementia care for migrants and refugees. As a result, no specific boundary was set on the date range of publication, and any relevant article was included in the literature review regardless of its publication date. Articles that were published in English were only included in the search. The keywords used for the literature search were "migrants," "cultural barrier," and "dementia support program," and these search terms were used to explore the cultural barriers faced by migrants in order to access dementia support programs. "Immigrants," "refugees," and "new comers" were also used within the keyword set as migrated population contains immigrants, newcomers, and refugee subgroups. Both "dementia" and "Alzheimer" research related to support programs and care designed for dementia and Alzheimer's disease are often comparable in nature and content, and frequently these two words were used interchangeably. Research regarding both support programs and care services are included in the literature review to encompass all types of barriers faced in regard to access to dementia care and support programs. Research conducted on populations including persons living with dementia, informal and formal caregivers (such as nurses, personal support workers, and other service providers), and dementia program facilitators and coordinators were included in the literature review. Research about barriers to equitable access among certain subgroups such as indigenous people was excluded from this review. Despite the diverse cultural background of indigenous population, this subgroup is not considered migrants.

2.2 Search strategy and data analysis

An extensive search of the literature was performed using the University of Ontario Institute of Technology (UOIT) library databases, including the PubMed databases and Wiley Library. The search strategy was consistent for every database and was based on the predetermined set of inclusion and exclusion criteria. Only full-text papers published in peer-reviewed journals and proceedings were selected for further review. Editorials, letters, and conceptual papers were excluded. All papers that addressed the keywords and search terms that were relevant to the research topic of interest were retrieved, regardless of their study design.

A total of 4451 research publications resulted from the keyword search from both databases which included peer-reviewed journal articles, eBooks/books, dissertations/thesis, and book chapters. Abstracts that were identified to be relevant to the research question were kept, and full-text papers were retrieved for further review. In the absence of an abstract, full-text papers were retrieved and reviewed for prospective inclusion. Reference lists of selected papers were examined to identify other relevant articles. There were a total of 15 articles included in the final data analysis using a thematic analysis method based on its relevance and the scope of research for data extraction purposes. The data extraction details about these 15 articles are presented in Appendix A. The findings were analyzed and synthesized to identify common themes, methodologies, and research gaps. In addition to the scholarly literature, gray literature found in credible websites were used to obtain information and findings such as statistical data, current approaches, and recommendations from the Alzheimer Society of Canada, Alzheimer's Society of the United Kingdom, and Statistics Canada.

3. Results and discussion

3.1 Key findings from literature review

Analysis of the existing literature that explored the underlying factors associated with the access to dementia support programs among migrant and refugee populations from diverse cultural backgrounds has led to the emergence of the following four themes, which are discussed below.

3.1.1 Stigma associated with dementia

The most common and impactful factor associated with the access to dementia support programs among migrants was stigma. The Alzheimer's Society of Ireland (2008) reported on two types of stigma, one as external, indicating stigma toward the person by community members, and the other as internal, indicating perceived feelings of shame about themselves that they are "less of a person" because of the symptoms of dementia [16]. Stigma affects the individual with dementia, which includes but is not limited to willingness to seek diagnosis and to seek support once diagnosed and a lack of willingness to participate in research [16]. In some cases, stigma about mental health impairments such as dementia was so deeply rooted that individuals and family members would deny to "recognize the illness" [17]. Data obtained from persons with dementia and family members reported that stigma often prevented them from seeking necessary information or support as "people would gossip about you if something went wrong" and "people don't want to get branded as odd or weird" [17].

In South Asian culture, mental health impairments including dementia are associated with perceived stigma toward the individual and their family members. A great deal of stigma appears to be associated with mental illness in such cultures where open discussion of a relative's mental health issues could cause the family to be stigmatized, with a reduced social standing that could affect later generations, such as interfering with marriage arrangements [15]. South Asian migrants thus appeared to be engaged in "concealment" as a mechanism to protect the reputation of the person with dementia and reputation of their family [15, 18]. The most common explanation for not using any support services among informal caregivers was that seeking support from outside agencies "put an already precarious balance between shame and inner pride in jeopardy" [18]. In Eastern European cultures, stigma associated with dementia also reinforces the tendency to "keep it in the family" instead of seeking support [18] as "going public" about having a family member with dementia is linked with a perceived fear of inviting condemnation from others in the community [18]. This reinforces the behavior of informal caregivers around providing support alone instead of seeking help from social and community support networks.

Persons with dementia were also identified to be vulnerable to experience stigma associated with chronic and severe mental illness, such as schizophrenia, because they shared a set of similar behavioral symptoms including depression, delusions, hallucinations, and agitation. For instance, researchers from Hong Kong outlined the social consequences of stigma associated with mental illness among Asian culture [19]. Lee and colleagues identified that concealment and anticipated stigmatization had a significant impact on non-compliance with care-seeking behavior. Persons with dementia and their family members attempted to hide their diagnosis from the community and forbid further interaction between the person with the illness and community members in the attempt to hide any shameful incidence [19]. Among Asian Americans such as Chinese and Vietnamese, shame and "loss of face" were identified to contribute to stigmatization associated with dementia [20] where shame was triggered by public display of abnormal behavior. Concealment was adopted to deflect such situations [21], resulting in delays and nonadherence to acquiring external care and support.

3.1.2 Culturally preferred coping strategies

Culturally preferred coping strategies were most prominent in South Asian immigrants and refugees where this specific characteristic reflected the ascribed stigma as discussed above. In fact, religion and culturally preferred coping strategies were identified to be particularly important within South Asian communities, opposed to the value of understanding symptom management and access to available resources, which is observed more in other ethnic minority groups [15]. South Asian subgroups appear to place high value on family where providing care for a family member is associated with the perception of responsibility toward their loved ones. In some South Asian cultures, "caring" was identified to be a religious obligation regardless of the religion, where caring was perceived as "duty" or a way of "gaining blessings" or "repaying" the person with dementia for previous acts of kindness [18]. Thus, South Asians have been reported to prefer providing care for a family member with a mental illness rather than seeking medical care, social care, or community support and assistance [15], leading to reduced engagement in dementia support programs or other social/medical care supports. Some South Asian subgroups were observed to use "faith" as an alternative coping strategy where faith is perceived to be associated with enhancing mental resilience and alleviation of stress experienced by persons with mental illnesses such as dementia and their caregivers [15]. Meditation and prayers were identified as tools used in religiously preferred coping strategies. The ideology of "caring" was also observed among Asian American migrants in addition to South Asian migrants. A study conducted on Korean immigrants with dementia revealed a concept of "Korean way of thinking," where caring for ill elderly in the family is considered a responsibility and is associated with "saving face" [22].

The concept of "acculturation" also appears as an important concept in terms of implications for support services among migrants. Acculturation varied depending on the length of stay in a migrated country and historical time of migration [22, 23]. Adoption of a foreign culture appears to be a selective process where fundamental values and beliefs appear to stay unchanged after immigration [22]. A study conducted on Korean immigrants in America indicated that those who migrated recently are more "Americanized" than those that migrated a long time ago and tend to preserve their traditional beliefs [22]. Failure to adopt the foreign culture can lead to the preservation of conventional norms and methods of practice in one's culture when dealing with chronic diseases, such as dementia.

3.1.3 Misconception regarding aging and Dementia

"Normalization" of functional and cognitive decline among older adult populations is observed to be a vastly shared belief in many cultures. Studies reveal that populations from ethnic minorities are less likely to recognize symptoms of dementia as an illness than Caucasian individuals, perceiving such symptoms as part of the aging process [24]. Normalization is observed among Asians, African-Caribbeans, and Hispanic Americans where dementia symptoms such as memory loss, disorientation, and loss of functional abilities were recognized but not conceptualized as an illness [25]. In Asian culture, dementia related to changes such as confusion is often normalized and expected as part of the aging process [20]. A majority of the common symptoms of dementia are interpreted as "age-related cognitive and functional change." Symptoms such as "memory failure" or "confusion" are considered normal among "very old" members of the family. Interviews conducted on subgroups originating from Chinese and Vietnamese cultures identified a culturally shaped metaphor that emphasized holism and the inevitability of deterioration in dementia [20], reinforcing the lack of understanding regarding the necessity of accessing dementia support programs.

Evidence from South Asian subgroups residing in England has identified that people from South Asian culture may recognize the symptoms associated with dementia but not conceptualize these as part of an illness even when they are severe [17], leading to the idea that individual and family efforts are sufficient to ameliorate dementia-related symptoms. Research conducted on South Asian families recognizes a generalized picture of aging that exists in South Asian culture where it is perceived that aging changes older people into an "intolerant and worrying" group and aging makes people "difficult and angry" [17]. Many dementia-related symptoms such as confusion, becoming quiet and sad, feelings of isolation and loneliness, and other mental health impairments are often viewed as "negative" aspects of normal aging [17, 24] in South Asian families. This leads to the conceptualization of not viewing dementia as an illness and therefore creating a barrier to accessing the external resources that support living well with dementia.

Another common misconception that exists in many different cultures is the lack of understanding on the causation of dementia. Dementia is often perceived as a mental illness by certain South Asian groups who are especially sensitive to traditional, religious, and spiritual explanations of the nature and causation of dementia [18]. Many South Asian cultures lack a defined vocabulary to interpret the word "dementia"; thus cases of dementia are often classified as a mental illness [15, 18]. Many individuals from South Asian cultures residing in the United Kingdom classify dementia as "madness" as the meaning of dementia is nonexistent in the vocabulary of South Asian languages [23]. In such cases, family members and the community at large frequently use concealment for avoiding rejection, which acts as an obstacle to accessing dementia support programs.

3.1.4 Language barrier

Language barrier was a significant factor leading to the reduced access to dementia support programs and services. Current literature revealed that migrants and refugees who do not speak the language of the host country might be at a greater disadvantage in accessing the health-care system [23], making the individual with a lack of language proficiency more vulnerable to inequitable access to dementia support services. Language difficulties often appear in Alzheimer's disease and other neurodegenerative dementias with word-finding difficulties, decreased verbal fluency, or difficulties with naming and comprehension, which are particularly prominent among bilingual individuals [26]. Older bilinguals often revert to a single language despite a lifetime of dual language use, losing the ability to speak the second language [26]. This issue is particularly prominent among migrants and refugees with dementia who lose their ability to speak their second languages, which is often the language of their host country, leading to difficulty in communicating with the health-care professionals and service providers [27]. Bilingual individuals with dementia are frequently observed to be inclined to asymmetrical language impairment with preferential preservation and the use of the first acquired language [28], which can be inferred among individuals that have migrated to a foreign country that speaks a different language than one's country of emigration. Moreover, recently learned information is retained the least in the case of dementia, whereas information and memory that are more remote are often relatively preserved, leading to a regression toward the predominant use of the language learnt earlier in life or the first language [26, 28].

Evidence obtained from the study of immigrants in Sweden suggested that immigrants with dementia noticeably preferred music and television programs that had more familiarity, such as programs in their native language [27]. They were also more likely to participate and engage in dementia support programs and services where they could communicate in their native language [23, 26]. Research evidence from Korean Americans with dementia suggested that treatment and intervention programs designed to promote living well with dementia were observed to be more effective when using a familiar language or the native language of the individual [29]. Inability to communicate well in the language of the program due to losing the ability to speak one's second language has been identified as one of the leading issues among individuals with dementia, particularly among those who have migrated from a foreign country with a different language than the host country.

4. Implications and conclusion

The literature review revealed that the most common underlying factors that influence reduced participation and access to dementia care and support programs among immigrant and refugee populations were stigma, culturally preferred coping strategies, misconceptions regarding aging and dementia, and language barriers. In particular, coping strategies were significantly influenced by the stigma associated with dementia as most cultures preferred concealment to avoid being negatively labeled in the community [15]. Misconceptions regarding aging and normalization of dementia are a commonly observed phenomenon among the majority of the well-known cultures in Europe and North America [16].

Research conducted on sociocultural factors and access to dementia care is often conducted among caregivers as opposed to the persons with dementia themselves, where conclusions made regarding the needs of persons with dementia were obtained indirectly from their care partners, formal and informal caregivers, and service providers. The rationale behind this approach was largely due to the difficulty of conducting research on persons with dementia as a result of their levels of cognitive impairment. In particular, there is a lack of empirical evidence obtained directly from persons living with dementia among migrated and refugee populations. Moreover, majority of the existing research about dementia care were conducted in certain countries such as in Europe and Australia. Findings from North American settings focused mainly on the American immigrants with dementia. There is a lack of research about the influencing sociocultural factors and access to dementia care/support programs among Canadian migrants. Most research examined barriers to access related to geographical location, economic status, educational level, and knowledge of dementia/care. There is a lack of empirical evidence on the impact of how stigma, cultural background, and language influence appropriate access to dementia support programs among migrants. There is also a lack of research that focuses on identifying the existing needs among immigrant populations with dementia in regard to their access to dementia care. These findings highlight the need to conduct further research on Canadian immigrants/refugees with dementia to further explore the key barriers faced by these populations in regard to accessing dementia care and support programs, as well as to identify the facilitating factors that meet the unique needs of Canadian migrants to promote living well with dementia.

Currently there are 564,000 Canadians living with dementia, and this number is doubling every 20 years [12, 30]. In addition to the rising number of persons with dementia, there has been a shift in the population triangle of Canada, with an increasing number of the population reaching the age 65 and up, which is the most vulnerable stage of life to develop dementia [30]. In particular, migratory increase has been identified as the major driving force of population growth in Canada, which indicates a change in the composition of the population with an increased cultural diversity [31]. As a result, it is imperative to increase our understanding of the influence of sociocultural factors in relation to equitable access of dementia care and support programs among the Canadian migrants. This knowledge is vital to the future transformation of the existing programs and services, shaping them to be more culturally inclusive for the marginalized, migrated, and refugee populations in Canada.

Competing interests

The authors declare that they have no competing interests.

Author's contributions

All authors provided input into the development of the literature review and have read and approved this manuscript.

Funding

The authors declare that there is no funding support for this project.

Ethical approval and consent to participate

Not applicable.

Appendix A. Summary of research studies included in the literature review

Author (date)	Study purpose	Study design	Summary of key findings
Swaffer K (2014)	Exploring the language being used to represent people with dementia, and the presence of stigma to identify if presence of stigma toward people with dementia aggravates the stigma or prevents the timely translation of good research into better practice	Robust literature review	• Stigma affects several aspects when considering dementia, including the person's willingness to seek diagnosis, to seek support once diagnosed, and a lack of willingness to participate in research • Caregiver stigma has been explored often but very little on the stigma as experienced directly by people with dementia

Author (date)	Study purpose	Study design	Summary of key findings
			• The language used in the current literature and the media and in the community creates an incorrect portrayal of persons living with the symptoms of dementia and creates and supports further stigmas and misconceptions regarding experience living with dementia. This eventually abolishes the value of the expression of the lived experiences, adding to the disbelief and stigma
Fontaine et al. (2007)	Explore the perceptions of aging, dementia, and aging-associated mental health difficulties among British people of Punjabi Indian origin	A focus group study was conducted between 2001 and 2003, involving 49 British South Asian individuals speaking English, Hindi, and Punjabi, aged 17–61 years. Data was collected on views of aging and aging-associated difficulties in initial groups. Following primary data collection, vignettes were used for more specific exploration of awareness and understanding of dementia in a second set of groups. Thematic analysis method was adopted to analyze data	• Perception of aging was as a time of withdrawal and isolation, and frequently mentioned health problems involved physical or emotional and cognitive impairment • Identified implications that symptoms of dementia partly resulted from lack of effort by the person themselves and possibly from lack of family care; thus overcoming own problems and family actions might be part of the solution • A sense of stigma and a lack of knowledge were identified about mental illness and services, along with disillusionment with doctors and exclusion from services
Giebel et al. (2015)	Examining the barriers and facilitators in accessing to culturally appropriate mental health care among South Asian older adults with memory impairment, dementia, and mental illness	A literature search was conducted in Web of Knowledge, PubMed, and Ovid databases to search for literatures from 1984 to 2012 regarding South Asian older adults or their family carers, their understandings	The following factors were identified by South Asians and health professionals that prevented help seeking and access to care: a lack of knowledge of dementia and mental illness and of local services, stigma, culturally

Author (date)	Study purpose	Study design	Summary of key findings
		of mental illness and dementia, and their pattern of service use. Assessment of abstracts for relevance and three researchers rated the quality of each included study. A narrative synthesis was used to extract and chart data	preferred coping strategies, and linguistic and cultural barriers in communication and decision-making
MacKenzie J (2006)	Summarize findings from a 3-year project to develop and deliver culturally appropriate support group materials for South Asian and Eastern European family carers of relatives with dementia living in the United Kingdom	Stage 1 involved semi-structured interviews for 21 participants to explore carers' experiences of caregiving. Stage 2 involved developing and delivering of three 10-week support group programs, specified to reflect the needs of carers (identified in Stage 1) in a range of preferred community languages. Follow-up interview was conducted in stage 3 with each of the family carers 6 weeks after the completion of group program	Understandings of dementia in different cultural contexts can become operationalized through stigma processes, thus influencing the ways in which person with dementia and their family carers' participation in formal and informal support programs
Lee et al. (2005)	Identify and compare the interpersonal experiences of stigma in patients with mental health impairments, schizophrenia, and diabetes mellitus in Hong Kong	Four focus groups were conducted to develop a self-report questionnaire. Data were collected from outpatients	Stigma was more frequently experienced among people living with mental health impairment from family members, partners, friends, and colleagues than those living with diabetes
Liu et al. (2008)	Examining the relationship of stigma and dementia among Chinese and Vietnamese family caregivers	32 qualitative interviews were conducted among Chinese and Vietnamese family caregivers living in the USA to collect narrative data and identify key themes	Two sources of stigma were identified: the stigma of chronic and severe mental illness and a stigma reflecting negative stereotypes of aging or the elderlies. Chinese and Vietnamese cultural perceptions of normal aging accommodate different paths of aging, some more and some less desired. With regard to persons with dementia, a "normalized" but negative path of aging carried with it significant stigma that was distinct from but in addition to the stigma of chronic and severe mental illness
Yang and Kleinman (2008)	An analysis of how "face" is embodied in China to understand an articulation of how the social aspects of	Analysis of existing conceptual writings and empirical studies	Face—both moral and in particular social face—can be seen to function as forms of symbolic capital. Shame

Author (date)	Study purpose	Study design	Summary of key findings
	stigma might incorporate the moral standing defined within a local context		and “loss of face” were identified to lead to stigmatization associated with mental health impairments including dementia
Kong et al. (2009)	To identify and describe experiences of Korean immigrant caregivers regarding American nursing home placement of their non-English-speaking older relatives with dementia	Qualitative descriptive methods and qualitative content analysis using a total of 17 semi-structured interviews with 10 Korean immigrant family caregivers	The “Korean way of thinking” was identified to be a fundamental cultural belief about caregiving. Six major themes were identified: (a) I never thought about a nursing home; (b) if I think in a Korean way, I feel; (c) nursing home staff cannot communicate with; (d) my care recipient maintains Korean culture; (e) nursing home services are better than expected but; and (f) my care recipient is more vulnerable because of dementia
Iliffe and Manthorpe (2010)	Argue that sociocultural/ ethnical issues are applicable to all individuals with dementia, independent of apparent ethnicity, and that promotion of cultural competence in service provision should not be relegated to an ethnic minority agenda	Analysis of existing literature	The experience of accessing to support is associated with three key factors: 1. Language and literacy 2. Religious belief and cultural practices 3. Coping mechanism and social support 4. Protective factors
Bunn et al. (2012)	Evaluate the qualitative evidence regarding how individuals accommodate and adapt to the diagnosis of dementia and its immediate consequences, to guide practice	Systemic review of qualitative studies using 102 studies from PubMed, PsycINFO, Embase, CINAHL, and the British Nursing Index databases. Thematic analysis was conducted	Three overarching themes emerged from the study: (1) pathways through diagnosis, including its impact on identity, roles, and relationships; (2) resolving conflicts to accommodate a diagnosis, including the acceptability of support, focusing on the present or the future, and the use or avoidance of knowledge; and (3) strategies and support to minimize the impact of dementia
Mukadam et al. (2011)	Explore the factors due to which people from minority ethnic (ME) groups with dementia present later to specialist, diagnostic, and	Systemic review using three quantitative and ten qualitative studies	Barriers to accessing support for dementia included not conceptualizing dementia as an illness; believing dementia was a normal

Author (date)	Study purpose	Study design	Summary of key findings
	therapeutic dementia services		consequence of aging; thinking dementia had spiritual, psychological, physical health or social causes; feeling that caring for the person with dementia was a personal or family responsibility; experiences of shame and stigma within the community; believing there was nothing that could be done to help; and negative experiences of health-care services. Accessing to help was facilitated by recognition of dementia as an illness and knowledge about dementia. Minority of the ethnic groups face significant barriers to help seeking for dementia, often diagnosed in late stage
McMurtay et al. (2009)	To explore whether regression to a primary language may be associated with development of cognitive impairment and increased risk for development of dementia	Studying two cases of bilingual patients who presented with early symptoms of dementia after regression to their primary language	The cases described in the report support the hypothesis that an association may exist between regression to the use of primary language among bilinguals and poor cognitive performance and diagnosis of dementia
Rosendahl et al. (2016)	Explore and elaborate the experiences of family members and professional caregivers regarding the care provided to immigrants with dementia in group homes in Sweden	Exploratory, descriptive study with a qualitative approach was chosen using in-depth semi-structured interviews. Qualitative content analysis was conducted to analyze data	Three main categories were determined with seven subcategories. The first main category was a new living situation which included the following subcategories: adjusting to new living arrangements and expectations regarding activities and traditional food at the group home; the second main category, challenges in communication with the subcategories: limited communication between the immigrant with dementia and the Swedish-speaking nursing staff and the consequences of linguistic misunderstandings and varied communication in a common language; and the third main category, the role of the family member at the

Author (date)	Study purpose	Study design	Summary of key findings
			group home with the subcategories: a link to the healthy life story of the family member with dementia and an expert and interpreter for the nursing staff
Mendez et al. (1999)	Explore the linguistic state of bilingual individuals with dementia	Survey 51 patients who reported regular use of another language, as well as varying fluency in English, and who presented for an evaluation because of progressive memory or cognitive problems such as dementia	Despite patients' differences in educational level, age at acquisition of English, frequency of use, and baseline fluency in English, a greater preference of the patients for their original language and decreased conversation in English was reported by all participating caregivers. With regard to characterizing the errors made by patients, majority of caregivers stated a tendency for words and phrases from the mother language used within English conversational speech
Kim et al. (2014)	Explore the relationship between nursing assistants' communication style and behavioral symptoms of individuals with dementia, focused on Korean American older adults with dementia residing in nursing homes	Reviewing currently available studies using eight studies from PubMed, CINAHL, PsycINFO, and ProQuest Digital Dissertations databases	Utilization of familiar language can increase an intervention's effect to potentially reduce or prevent behavioral symptoms of dementia for immigrants from various countries

Author details

Winnie Sun[1*], Srija Biswas[1], Michelle Dacanay[1] and Ping Zou[2]

1 Faculty of Health Sciences, University of Ontario Institute of Technology, Oshawa, Canada

2 School of Nursing, Nipissing University, Toronto, Ontario, Canada

*Address all correspondence to: winnie.sun@uoit.ca

References

[1] Government of Canada, "Dementia," Government of Canada [Online]. 2016. Available from: https://www.canada.ca/en/public-health/services/diseases/dementia.html [Accessed: 28-03-2017]

[2] Alzheimer's Association. 2015 Alzheimer's disease facts and figures. Alzheimer's & Dementia. 2015;**11**(3): 332-384. Retrieved from: https://www.alz.org/facts/downloads/facts_figures_2015.pdf

[3] Statistics Canada. Seniors. 2016. Retrieved from: http://www.statcan.gc.ca/pub/11-402-x/2012000/chap/seniors-aines/seniors-aines-eng.htm

[4] Makwarimba E, Stewart M, Simich I, Makumbe K, Shizha E, Anderson S. Sudanese and Somali refugees in Canada: Social support needs and preferences. International Migration. 2013;**51**(5):106-119

[5] Scheltens P, Blennow K, Bretler MMB, de Strooper B, Frisoni GB, Salloway S, et al. Alzheimer's disease. Lancet. 2016;**338**(10043):505-517. DOI: 10.1016/S0140-6736(15)01124-1

[6] Wong SL, Gilmour H, Ramage-Morin PL. Health Reports: Alzheimer's Disease and other Dementias in Canada. Statistics Canada [Internet]. 2016. Available from: https://www.statcan.gc.ca/pub/82-003-x/2016005/article/14613-eng.htm. [Cited: 26-03-2018]

[7] Alzheimer Society of Canada. Normal Aging vs Dementia. Alzheimer Society of Canada [Internet]. 2017. Available from: http://alzheimer.ca/en/Home/About-dementia/What-is-dementia/Normal-aging-vs-dementia [Cited: 26-03-2018]

[8] Dubois B, Padovani A, Scheltens P, Rossi A, Dell'Agnello G. Timely diagnosis for Alzheimer's disease: A literature review on benefits and challenges. Journal of Alzheimer's Disease. 2016;**41**(3):617-631. DOI: 10.3233/JAD-150692

[9] Dementia in the Asia Pacific Region. Alzheimer's Disease International. 2014. Available from: https://www.alz.co.uk/dementia-in-the-asia-pacific

[10] Brodaty H, Donkin M. Family caregivers of people with dementia. Dialogues in Clinical Neuroscience. 2009;**11**(2):217-228

[11] Reinhard SC, Given B, Petlick NH, Bemis A. Supporting family caregivers in providing care. In: Patient Safety and Quality: An Evidence-Based Handbook for Nurses. Rockville: Agency for Healthcare Research and Quality; 2008

[12] Alzheimer Society Canada, "Dementia Numbers in Canada," Alzheimer Society Canada [Online] 2017. Available from: http://www.alzheimer.ca/en/About-dementia/what-is-dementia/Dementia-numbers [Accessed: 11-03-2017]

[13] Koehn S, Neysmith S, Kobayashi K, Khamisa H. Revealing the shape of knowledge using an intersectionality lens: Results of a scoping review on the health and health care of ethnocultural minority older adults. The International Journal of Aging and Society. 2013;**33**: 437-464

[14] Statistics Canada, "Population growth: Migratory increase overtakes natural increase," Statistics Canada [Online] 2017. Available from: http://www.statcan.gc.ca/pub/11-630-x/11-630-x2014001-eng.htm [Accessed: 25-03-2017]

[15] Giebel CM, Zubair M, Jolley D, Bhui KS, Challis D. South Asian older adults with memory impairment: Improving assessment and access to dementia care.

International Journal of Geriatric Psychiatry. 2014;**30**(4):345-356

[16] Swaffer k. Dementia: Stigma, language, and dementia-friendly. SAGE. 2014;**13**(6):709-716

[17] Fontaine JL, Ahuja J, Bradbury NM, Phillips S, Oyebode JR. Understanding dementia amongst people in minority ethnic and cultural groups. Journal of Advanced Nursing. 2007;**60**(6):605-614

[18] Mackenzie J. Stigma and dementia. Dementia. 2006;**5**(2):233-247

[19] Lee S, Lee MT, Chiu MY, Kleinman A. Experience of social stigma by people with schizophrenia in Hong Kong. British Journal of Psychiatry. 2005; **186**(2):153-157

[20] Liu D, Hinton L, Tran C, Hinton D, Barker JC. Reexamining the relationships among dementia, stigma and aging in immigrant Chinese and Vietnamese family caregivers. Journal of Cross-Cultural Gerontology. 2008;**23**: 283-299

[21] Yang LY, Klainman A. 'Face' and the embodiment of stigma in China: The cases of schizophrenia and AIDS. Social Science & Medicine. 2008;**67**(3):398-408

[22] Kong E-H, Deatrick JA, Evans LK. The experiences of Korean immigrant caregivers of non-English-speaking older relatives with dementia in American nursing homes. Qualitative Health Research. 2010;**20**(3):319-329

[23] Iliffe S, Manthorpe J. The debate on ethnicity and dementia: From category fallacy to person-centred care? Aging and Mental Health. 2004;**8**(4):283-292

[24] Bunn F, Goodman C, Sworn K, Rait G, Brayne C, Robinson L. Psychosocial factors that shape patient and carer experiences of dementia diagnosis and treatment: A systematic review of qualitative studies. PLoS Medicine. 2012;**9**(10)

[25] Mukadam N, Cooper C, Livingston G. A systematic review of ethnicity and pathways to care in dementia. International Journal of Geriatric Psychiatry. 2011;**26**:12-20

[26] McMurtay A, Saito E, Nakamoto B. Language preference and development of dementia among bilingual individuals. Hawaii Journal of Medicine & Public Health. 2009;**68**(9):223-226

[27] Rosendahl SP, Soderman M, Mazaheri M. Immigrants with dementia in Swedish residential care: An exploratory study of the experiences of their family members and nursing staff. BMC Geriatrics. 2016;**16**:18

[28] Mendz M, Perryman KM, Ponton MO, Jeffery CL. Bilingualism and dementia. The Journal of Neuropsychiatry and Clinical Neurosciences. 1999;**11**(3):411-412

[29] Kim H, Wood DL, Phillips LR. Nursing assistants' communication styles in Korean American older adults with dementia. Journal of Transcultural Nursing. 2014;**26**(2):185-192

[30] Wong SL, Gilmour H, Ramage-Morin PL. "Health Reports Alzheimer's Disease and other Dementias in Canada," Statistics Canada [Online] 2016. Available from: http://www.statcan.gc.ca/pub/82-003-x/2016005/article/14613-eng.htm [Accessed: 27-02-2017]

[31] Statistics Canada, "Population Growth: Migratory Increase Overtakes Natural Increase," Statistics Canada [Online] 2017. Available from: http://www.statcan.gc.ca/pub/11-630-x/11-630-x2014001-eng.htm [Accessed: 11-03-2017]